Foundations of
Problem-based Learning

SRHE and Open University Press Imprint
General Editor: Heather Eggins

Current titles include:

Foundations of Problem-based Learning

Maggi Savin-Baden and
Claire Howell Major

Society for Research into Higher Education
& Open University Press

Open University Press
McGraw-Hill Education
McGraw-Hill House
Shoppenhangers Road
Maidenhead
Berkshire
England
SL6 2QL

email: enquiries@openup.co.uk
world wide web: www.openup.co.uk

and Two Penn Plaza, New York, NY 10121-2289, USA

First published 2004

A catalogue record of this book is available from the British Library

ISBN 0 335 21531 9 (pb)   0 335 21532 7 (hb)

Library of Congress Cataloging-in-Publication Data
CIP data applied for

Typeset by RefineCatch Ltd, Bungay, Suffolk
Printed in Great Britain by MPG Books Ltd, Bodmin, Cornwall

To John and Ted, our supportive husbands.

Contents

Acknowledgements

Thanks are due to a number of people: Barbara Duch, Beth Jones, Karen O'Rourke, Betsy Palmer, Kay Sambell and Kay Wilkie for their helpful and critical comments on the text and Roy Cox for permission to use his figure in Chapter 13.

We are grateful to all those who have participated in our research over the last ten years and agreed to be quoted here. Our grateful thanks are also due to Bob Rankin for the design and permission to use the cartoon on the front cover.

Finally our thanks are due to John Savin-Baden for his support, patience, proofreading, critical sense of humour and for managing two challenging children while we wrote, and to Ted Major for supporting us amid career demands. The views expressed here and any errors are ours.

Prologue

We sat in a French café in Alabama, USA. We had never met before, yet we were colleagues. We knew each other's writing style and views on problem-based learning. Without formal introductions we launched comfortably into the middle of a conversation.

'So,' Claire said, in her careful yet distinct southern American English. 'What are we going to do about this yawning gap in the market? Who is writing a text that deals with the foundations of problem-based learning and is really coming to grips with the issues?'

'Not me,' I said, aware in my southern American surroundings of my British English. 'I am writing the stuff I hope will challenge current practice, books for the experienced, not the novices.'

'But this text is badly needed.' The meal arrived and we shared family photos and talked of our academic lives.

'Okay, let's write it,' I said, as Claire dropped me at the airport.

The virtual world is both a challenging and an interesting one. While the virtual world sometimes breeds difficulties in communicating clearly, without it, communication might not be possible in the first place. At its best, the virtual world is one in which globalization becomes a reality, a place where it is possible to transcend the boundaries of our physical locations and a place where scholars with shared interests can exchange ideas and information.

It was in this world that Claire and I interacted and worked together for over three years before we met face to face. We had used e-mail, written papers together, edited a journal and felt that we had done all right. During these exchanges, we both suggested the need for a text that not only provided some sensible and down-to-earth suggestions about implementing problem-based learning and charted its history, but also looked at the influence of a number of agendas on problem-based learning. Neither of us thought, over the ether, of suggesting that we should write it together. Yet towards the end of 2002 we met in Birmingham, Alabama for lunch and decided to write this text.

Maggi: My experience of problem-based learning is largely based in my research and consultancy in the UK, although I visit and speak around the world. I enjoy using problem-based learning in my Master's teaching, but still I both struggle and delight in watching students come to terms with accepting they do have a stance and a voice. Many of the ideas and suggestions in this text have emerged from my consultancy work in the UK and Ireland and from those who have taken some of my more unconventional suggestions forward. My interest in models of curriculum design and problem-based learning curricula continues to grow. Yet most of the time I still feel that, like most things in this world, problem-based learning and higher education hold few straightforward answers. Problem-based learning, I believe, is a chance to learn with and through complexity.

Claire: My expertise is largely based in my US experience, despite my interactions with the international community. I came to problem-based learning initially as an academic developer, working with new staff members who wanted to implement problem-based learning in their programmes and courses. This work stimulated research activity as I began to examine shifting from traditional pedagogies, such as lecture and discussion, to implementing problem-based learning that demanded changes in tutors' pedagogical content knowledge (their thinking about the nature and structure of knowledge, curricula, students, learning, instructional techniques and generally about the best ways to teach in a specific discipline). I soon began to understand problem-based learning as a fundamental shift in philosophy and I currently use problem-based learning in my own teaching, understanding from a first-hand perspective what that philosophical change entails.

Our experiences with and interests in problem-based learning vary. However, what we would both argue is that the notion of learning through managing problems is not new, and it is possible to trace the origins of problem-based learning back to a variety of positions about the nature of learning and education, many of which we describe in this text.

   This book sets out to present the history of and changes in problem-based learning, explore traditional understandings of problem-based learning curricula and examine new and emerging issues. It suggests ways of dealing with some of the many concerns raised by tutors, such as designing problems, issues related to learning in teams and assessing learning. It also examines current challenges in the field, such as the need to embrace diversity and understand distributed learning, and proposes ways of preventing curricula drift away from problem-based learning. Through this book we argue that:

1   understanding the broad historical base of this approach to learning can help us to appreciate theoretical underpinnings of the method and how problem-based learning fits within a tutor's philosophical framework;
2   examining different curricula models can help us to re-evaluate our current programmes and explore the extent to which components from

other disciplines, curricula and models can help us improve our own programmes;

3 engaging with diverse debates about learning, assessment and teamwork can enable us to develop and refine our current approaches to teaching;

4 realizing that cultural diversity, academic agendas and governmental ideologies have a significant impact on our programmes and can enable us to be aware of the differences of our espoused and actual practices in problem-based learning.

The book is presented in three parts. Part 1 documents the philosophical, psychological, historical and cultural foundations of problem-based learning. Part 2 explores curricula issues including the position of teams, tutors and students in problem-based learning and how students should be assessed. Part 3 examines new and emerging concerns and considers the need for new and different forms of research, including evaluation, to be undertaken in this field.

Part 1, entitled 'Conceptual frames', contains an overview of the emergence of problem-based learning globally and maps its growth. Chapter 1 explores the philosophical and epistemological concepts underpinning problem-based learning and continues with a consideration of the early developments in, and varieties of, problem-based learning. Chapter 2 provides a historical overview of the beginnings and later development of problem-based learning globally and analyses the reasons for its emergence and continuing popularity. Chapter 3 begins with an exploration of the impacts that behavioural, cognitive, developmental and humanistic theories have had on problem-based learning. It then presents theories that focus on the value of meaning construction, personal transition, learning context and learner identity. In Chapter 4, we present new work on curricula models that explores how problem-based learning actually occurs in practice, and we examine the impact of such modes of curriculum practice from the point of view of students, staff and institutions. Chapter 5 explores understandings of culture and in particular the different dimensions of national, disciplinary and institutional cultures that influence problem-based learning. It concludes by considering the types of leadership necessary to overcome cultural barriers.

Part 2 is the applied area of the book that explores some of the concerns about the realities of implementing problem-based learning. These chapters are based strongly on the experience of the authors, as both researchers of and consultants in problem-based learning. Thus many of the issues discussed here first emerged as questions from participants in problem-based learning workshops around the world. In Chapter 6 we examine what might count as a problem and explore some of the literature that relates to this. We suggest that it is important to consider how problems are used in a course or programme and that problems should be designed not only so that students use different types of knowledge and capabilities but also so that they motivate and keep motivating students. The issue of learning in teams is an area that has received increasing attention since the late 1980s and in Chapter 7 we outline some of the advantages and characteristics of team learning and suggest ways of creating successful teams. In Chapter 8 we explore the shift in role that students face when they move from the traditional teaching situation to the problem-based learning environment and discuss the range of student roles and responsibilities that students face in problem-based learning. Chapters 9 and 10 explore issues relating to the role of tutors in problem-based learning and argue that equipping them for this approach is still an area of much debate. These chapters examine the recent research in these areas and suggest practical ways of engaging with some of the difficulties. The final chapter in this section then explores the impact of assessment on problem-based learning.

Part 3 concludes the book by exploring some of the new and emerging trends in problem-based learning and is designed to help the reader to consider a number of decisions that need to be taken on the road to implementation, as well as during and after implementation, in order that it can be sustained. Chapter 12 explores issues of diversity, in terms of student experience, ability, background, race and culture. It also examines recent research into using problem-based learning with non-dominant cultures. Chapter 13 examines ways of evaluating programmes that have adopted problem-based learning and explores the evidence for their effectiveness. Chapter 14 examines the research and practice of sustaining problem-based learning at a staff and institutional level, exploring such areas as ongoing support for facilitators, development of new staff and curriculum development. The epilogue suggests some of the changes that need to be addressed both with and beyond the problem-based learning community while arguing for the importance and need to reposition the place of electronic and distance learning in relation to problem-based learning.

This is a book that we hope will not only provide guidance to those wanting to implement problem-based learning, but will also provoke debate in the problem-based learning community, about such subjects as curriculum design, the position of assessment, the value of working in teams, and issues of power and control in the learning process. Such foundational concerns are ones that we believe are vital for underpinning sound problem-based learning with a critical edge.

Part I

Conceptual frames

1
Delineating core concepts of problem-based learning

Introduction

In this chapter, we introduce the problem-based learning approach and identify some of the leading debates that surround it. We examine the method's core elements and key characteristics. In our analysis of problem-based learning and the changes it has undergone over time, we argue that flexibility and diversity are vital to ensure that through problem-based learning both students and tutors come to own and value their shifts and transitions in learning. Thus, for many, problem-based learning might be seen as an ideology rooted in the experiential learning tradition that can be adopted within modules, across semesters or throughout curricula.

Early definitions of problem-based learning

Compared with many pedagogical approaches problem-based learning has emerged relatively recently, being popularized by Barrows and Tamblyn (1980) following their research into the reasoning abilities of medical students at McMaster Medical School in Canada. Barrows and Tamblyn's study and the approach adopted at McMaster marked a clear move away from problem-solving learning in which individual students answer a series of questions from information supplied by a lecturer. Rather, this new method they proposed involved learning in ways that used problem scenarios to encourage students to engage themselves in the learning process, a method to become known as *problem-based learning*.

In this early version of problem-based learning certain key characteristics were essential. Students in small teams[1] would explore a problem situation and through this exploration were expected to examine the gaps in their own knowledge and skills in order to decide what information they needed to acquire in order to resolve or manage the situation with which they were presented. Thus, early definitions of problem-based learning identify the classic model as one that has the following characteristics (Barrows and Tamblyn 1980):

- Complex, real world situations that have no one 'right' answer are the organizing focus for learning.
- Students work in teams to confront the problem, to identify learning gaps, and to develop viable solutions.
- Students gain new information though self-directed learning.
- Staff act as facilitators.
- Problems lead to the development of clinical problem-solving capabilities.

Expanding the themes

Problem-based learning has expanded world-wide since the 1960s, and as it has spread the concepts associated with it have changed and become more flexible and fluid than in former years. In an attempt to move beyond narrow and prescriptive definitions Boud (1985) and Barrows (1986), two of the stronger proponents of the approach, have outlined broader characteristics of problem-based learning. Both have argued that problem-based learning is not to be seen as a particular way or method of learning; rather it is to be seen as learning that has a number of differing forms. Boud (1985) suggested that problem-based learning differs according to the nature of the discipline and the particular goals of the programme. He noted that developments in problem-based learning have drawn on a number of ideas in addition to problem-centredness, the most important of which he sees as student-centredness. Boud outlined eight other characteristics of many problem-based learning courses:

1   an acknowledgement of the base of experience of learners;
2   an emphasis on students taking responsibility for their own learning;
3   a crossing of boundaries between disciplines;
4   an intertwining of theory and practice;
5   a focus on the processes rather than the products of knowledge acquisition;
6   a change in the tutor's role from that of instructor to that of facilitator;
7   a change in focus from tutors' assessment of outcomes of learning to student self-assessment and peer assessment;
8   a focus on communication and interpersonal skills so that students understand that in order to relate their knowledge, they require skills to communicate with others, skills that go beyond their area of technical expertise.

These characteristics mark a distinct shift from the earlier, more rigid definitions of problem-based learning that focus on what goes on during a session; rather Boud's characteristics elaborate on the pedagogical beliefs underlying the approach.

Varieties in approach

Barrows has suggested that the combination of design variables for problem-based learning, when linked to the educational objectives, is endless. He concluded that the term problem-based learning must be considered a genus from which there are many species and subspecies. As such, all types of problem-based learning must be evaluated in terms of issues such as the type of problems, assessment methods, learners' autonomy and the way in which teaching and learning occurs. Barrows (1986) thus proposed a taxonomy of problem-based learning methods that explains differing meanings and uses of problem-based learning. The taxonomy has highlighted the educational objectives that it is possible to address through problem-based learning and has included the following combination of varieties in use:

1   Lecture-based cases: here students are presented with information through lectures and then case material is used to demonstrate that information.
2   Case-based lectures: in this instance students are presented with case histories or vignettes before a lecture that then covers relevant material.
3   Case method: students are given a complete case study that must be researched and prepared for discussion in the next class.
4   Modified case-based: here students are presented with some information and are asked to decide on the forms of action and decisions they may make. Following their conclusions, they are provided with more information about the case.
5   Problem-based: in this instance students meet with a client in some form of simulated format that allows for free inquiry to take place.
6   Closed-loop problem-based: this is an extension of the problem-based method, where students are asked to consider the resources they used in the process of problem solving in order to evaluate how they may have reasoned through the problem more effectively.

The perspectives offered by Barrows and Boud have demonstrated the multifaceted nature of problem-based learning.

Broadening the philosophy

Since the popularization of problem-based learning, many have continued the attempt to define it in some way, and thus the stances developed by Barrows and Boud have been supported and subsequently developed by many (Margetson 1991; Savin-Baden 2000; Duch *et al.* 2001). Walton and Matthews (1989), for example, have argued that problem-based learning is to be understood as a general educational strategy or even as a philosophy rather than merely as a teaching approach. They believe that there is no fixed agreement as to what does and does not constitute problem-based learning. However they have argued that for problem-based learning to be present, three components must be able to be differentiated. The suggestion that these authors make offers clarity about how problem-based learning might be seen and understood. What they offer are parameters within which to understand problem-based learning without losing the sense of its vitality and complexity as an approach. The three broad areas of differentiation are as follows:

- essential characteristics of problem-based learning that comprised curricula organization around problems rather than disciplines, an integrated curriculum and an emphasis on cognitive skills;
- conditions that facilitated problem-based learning such as small groups, tutorial instruction, and active learning;
- outcomes that were facilitated by problem-based learning such as the development of skills and motivation, together with the development of the ability to be life-long learners.

This particular interpretation of problem-based learning offers a way of understanding this educational strategy that takes account of the complex nature of learning. At the same time it is an interpretation that encapsulates the differing ways in which students learn in diverse professions and disciplines across a variety of institutions.

Blurred edges?

Merely to list specific and narrowly defined characteristics does not in fact untangle the philosophical conundrums of problem-based learning. Rather than describing characteristics such as those provided by Boud or typologies as delineated by Barrows, there has been a shift towards understanding that problem-based learning is one of many active approaches to learning that make student learning and self-direction central components. Indeed, the number and variety of approaches to active learning has increased during the past few decades in a response to the growing dissatisfaction with the traditional teacher-centred paradigm. This has occurred too at a time when there has been an increasing focus by government and professions on what it is that students are able to *do* as a result of a university education. Such demands have not only resulted in pressure to change but have also put issues of how students learn in higher education centre stage. Forms of problem-based learning have evolved to reflect such change, and this has resulted in confusion about the different types on offer. For this reason, we differentiate some of the differences between these approaches in Table 1.1.

We are now facing such diversity in the field of problem-based learning along with confusions about the interrelationship between problem-based learning, project-based learning, problem-solving learning, action learning and work-based learning, that advocates of problem-based learning are often becoming prescriptive in an attempt to differentiate it. We do not intend

Table 1.1 Comparison of forms of active learning

Method	Organization of knowledge	Forms of knowledge	Role of student	Role of tutor	Type of activity
Problem-based learning	Open-ended situations and problems	Contingent and constructed	Active participants and independent critical inquirers who own their own learning experiences	Enabler of opportunities for learning	Development of strategies to facilitate team and individual learning
Project-based learning	Tutor-set, structured tasks	Performative and practical	Completer of project or member of project team who develops a solution or strategy	Task setter and project supervisor	Problem solving and problem management
Problem-solving learning	Step-by-step logical problem-solving through knowledge supplied by lecturer	Largely propositional but may also be practical	Problem solver who acquires knowledge through bounded problem solving	A guide to the right knowledge and solution	Finding solutions to given problems
Action learning	Group-led discussion and reflection on action	Personal and performative	Self-adviser who seeks to achieve own goals and help others achieve their's through reflection and action	A facilitator of reflection and action	Achievement of individual goals

to join the prescriptive camp; rather we intend to be more analytical than prescriptive. However, we would also argue that clarity in the underlying purpose of the approach and clarity of the students' and tutors' positions within the approach can facilitate effective learning. To support our position by way of an example, we offer the following incident. We recently had lunch with a senior university manager who argued that students did not need to be informed about what type of learning they were doing. For him the differences in the aims did not matter, as long as the students were learning rather than just having their heads filled with knowledge. However, we argued that if students are to be self-directed learners who are expected to take control of their learning and understand the context in which they learn best, then they need to understand the differences in approaches and the relative amount of freedom that one would seem to offer over another. Arguably the tutor, the university and even the country will affect this, but we believe such information is vital for students so that they can own their learning experiences and become independent in inquiry.

Conclusion

Since its inception, interest has grown in problem-based learning and such growth can be seen in the number of curricula and modules that now adopt it as their guiding principle. The surge in interest is perhaps due to the promise that it seems to hold for helping us to achieve our multiple and often divergent educational goals. However, the approach is not without challenges, not least because of the confusion about its relationship with other forms of action-orientated learning. For us, there are no narrowly defined characteristics of problem-based learning. Instead there are people working in contexts using problem-based approaches. Problem-based learning is an approach to learning that is affected by the structural and pedagogical environment into which it is placed, in terms of the discipline or subject, the tutors and the organization concerned. Our approach in investigating and reporting on this method is thus analytical rather than prescriptive. While we acknowledge that problem-based learning is undergoing a massive process of change world-wide, such change has been analysed by few in the field of higher education. By beginning to outline the theoretical constructs of the method and how they have changed over time, we believe that we have set the stage for the remainder of this book.

Note

1   The word team is used throughout the book to denote a group of people who work together with a common purpose, have a limited membership and the power to make decisions. Teams have a focus, a set of team rules and are time limited. The term team is more appropriate than group to denote what occurs in

most problem-based learning seminars because there is a focus, a remit and much of the learning that occurs evolves through the ways in which the team make decisions about what and how they learn within agreed or contracted deadlines.

2

A brief history of problem-based learning

Introduction

The notion of learning through solving problems is not new, and the emergence and development of problem-based learning through a history of ideas over time is marked by change. The twentieth century was an era marked by criticism as well as increased calls for accountability in higher education, particularly in the area of teaching and learning. Internationally, educators began to question traditional teaching methods where the staff member acts as the primary vehicle of information. The development of knowledge began to be viewed as a process through which individuals must grapple with complex questions, conduct original investigations and filter information through their social and cultural contexts. The negotiation of meaning, the focus on experience and the development of sound social practices and ideologies began to be viewed as central to the exploration of the nature of knowledge. As these ideas converged with other contextual forces, space opened for change, and problem-based learning emerged as an innovative approach to education.

Epistemological origins of problem-based learning

Problem-based learning has origins in a number of schools of philosophical thought, as changes in understandings about the nature of knowledge gave rise to educational approaches designed to help people acquire or develop it. We discuss a range of many of these epistemological origins below.

Connections with naturalism: developing knowledge through questioning

One of the primary features of problem-based learning is that it enables students to question the nature of a problem and consider how it might best be investigated, an aspect that draws from early philosophical notions, dating back as far as the seventh century BC philosophy of the Milesians, or Ionians, which included the works of Thales, Anaximander and Anaxagoras. Such philosophers explored cosmological questions such as, 'What is the original matter of which the bodily world is made?' This group sought to define the ultimate nature of things by positing a single word as the principle for explaining the deeper meaning of things. While not an enduring philosophy, this school of thought did have several lasting influences on our conception of how people gain knowledge. The Milesians, for example, advocated a questioning approach to develop understanding and in this way helped shape the beginning of a critical questioning approach to learning.

Connections with metaphysics: critiquing knowledge through reason

Problem-based learning is an approach in which it is acknowledged that learners should develop metacognitive skills and thus it is expected that students use reasoning abilities to manage or solve complex problems. These ideas also date back to ancient Greek philosophers, when in the fifth and fourth century BC the Sophists became the first to consider the epistemological question, 'What is the nature and reliability of human knowledge?' These notions connect closely with problem-based learning that takes at its core the idea that knowledge is personal. Later the Sceptics in this tradition questioned human ability to know, avoided doctrines and dogmas, sought to criticize existing ideas and believed that the human mind was incapable of taking in knowledge without distorting whatever it perceived or conceived. The Sceptics claimed that truth and knowledge were all relative to the individual or the group and that there were no valid absolutes, a claim consistent with the philosophical tenets of problem-based learning.

The metaphysical perspective peaked during the fifth and fourth century BC, when the trio of Socrates, Plato and Aristotle fundamentally changed views of knowledge acquisition. Socrates, the first of these famous Greek philosophers, believed that knowledge is unattainable. To prove his claim, he used dialogue and questioning approaches to probe student understanding of moral concepts such as justice, and applied formal logic to their ideas to show inconsistencies, inadequacies and weaknesses of their beliefs. He wanted students to think harder and search to discover truth within themselves. His method evolved into the current notion of the Socratic method or Socratic dialogue. This questioning and probing of assumptions and beliefs is inherent in problem-based learning, where it is used to help students question their knowledge when they confront new problems.

Plato, who studied under Socrates and followed in his mentor's footsteps, was not as entrenched in his beliefs that knowledge was unattainable. Plato instead centred on the use of idealism, or what is real is what we can reason, to develop understanding. Knowledge according to Plato could not be gained through sensory perceptions alone; rather, knowledge must also involve a form of intuition. He also founded the Academy, perhaps one of the first formal institutions of learning. Plato believed that learning should not be forced and that lessons should come in the form of play (Plato, *Republic*). In problem-based learning, students use intuition to solve problems in a simulated context.

Problem-based learning requires students to gain information through sensory perception as well as by using logic. This notion can be traced back to Aristotle who focused on realism and believed that the real could exist independent of the senses and that knowledge could be gained through perception as well as by abstraction and logical reasoning. Thus Aristotle trained students in the dialectic, in which students tried to reconcile oppositions presented in a thesis or problem. In the Aristotelian teaching act, the teacher instructed a learner about some object, some body of knowledge or some discipline. Teaching and learning never represented merely an interpersonal relationship or the expression of feelings; rather, they were always about disciplined inquiry into some aspect of reality. Education should cultivate and develop each person's rationality, enable students to make rational judgements on many subjects and serve the theoretical and practical by combining technical skills, liberal education, subjects and theory. These notions connect with problem-based learning as students attempt to develop knowledge, engage in sustained inquiry and seek to develop practical skills. This Greek trio left educators with the legacy of examination, inquiry and questioning, as well as an understanding of knowledge as something that is imprecise at best and shaped by the knower.

Connections with rationalism: deductive reasoning to examine impressions

Rationalism assumes that humans do not know things directly but grasp only their impressions, thus phenomena is concerned with the impressions made on the intellect. Rationalism adopted a model of mathematical deduction. This strand of thought is best known in the works of the seventeenth-century philosopher, Descartes, who perhaps best captured it in the phrase 'I think, therefore I am.' However, his views do still influence and reinforce the divide between mind and matter and intellect and emotion. Problem-based learning connects with this philosophical tradition through its emphasis on deductive reasoning as students examine and solve a problem, but unlike rationalist discourse it would seek to encourage strong links between intellect and emotions.

Connections with empiricism: scientific observation and discovery

Problem-based learning requires students to solve complex problems through sustained inquiry and investigation using inductive as well as deductive reasoning to come to a solution. These notions date back to the emergence of modern philosophy with the empirical tendency as espoused by Bacon, Hobbes, Locke, Berkeley and Hume, whose philosophical approach accepts sensory experience as a source of knowledge. Bacon and Locke challenged rationalism in the seventeenth century by proposing that the source of knowledge must be the observable environment rather than innate ideas or premises. Thus empiricism developed along with the emergence of the scientific method. Empiricists posit that observable reality is the undistorted picture of the world, and that knowledge comes from our inductive reasoning of the evidence received from experiences and observations. Thus we gain knowledge from gathering information and from testing our understanding of experience with the external world.

Connections with phenomenologicalism: individual perception of knowledge

Problem-based learning is designed to connect knowledge learned in academe with knowledge needed for the workplace. It gives students a space for trying out new ideas in safe environments. This traces to more modern philosophers such as Kant, who agreed with the Sceptics that we could not know reality, but we could only know the appearance of things. He argued (Kant 1983) that while both rational and empirical views require that the individuals go outside themselves in order to know the world, there is a different level of reality to consider. That level consists of how the world appears to the individual, or the phenomenological realm. We impose order and objectivity on experience that is dictated by the structure of our brains. In other words, as we interact with reality, we use temporal (categorization, listing, comparison/contrast) or spatial (cause/effect, sequence) dimensions to make meaning of our experiences and to construct knowledge. Kant believed that the physical world is not all there is. Thus, we can know how things seem to our minds but not how they really are. He believed that knowledge is a means to an end and that the end should benefit society. Kant is perhaps one of the first to identify a gap between theory or knowledge and practice, as he states, 'Between theory and practice, no matter how complete the theory may be, a middle term that provides a connection and transition is necessary' (Kant 1983: 61). Education should help negotiate that gap, and in a problem-based learning course it does.

Connections with positivism: notions of social justice emerge

Problem-based learning would seem to address many issues of social justice, as it provides students who may be otherwise marginalized in traditional classes with the opportunity to participate. The ideas of social justice have their origins in the last half of the nineteenth century, brought about by the broad movement of positivism. The positivists conceived of matter as a unique reality having the power of evolving from the lower to the higher forms. This evolution was even extended to include humans. Positivist philosophy consists in knowing the fundamental laws that govern matter in its process of evolution. The founder of positivism was Comte; its best and most systematic thinkers were English, and is apparent in the works of Bentham, James Mill and John Stuart Mill, who argued for utilitarian ideals and for the notion that education could fundamentally change lives and provide for political and social justice. A problem-based learning class is designed to reach all students, including those who might otherwise be marginalized. However, according to Popper (1970), all thought (and presumably action and experience) takes place within some kind of framework, although we are not forever confined to this framework. Barnett (1994) has argued that Popper avoided the issue that the practical rules of a particular framework forbid its examination. To do so would run counter to the very nature of the framework, because by deconstructing one framework that is the basis of the discipline, other related frameworks thereby become problematic as all the other connecting boundaries become problematic. Yet in problem-based learning students should, we suggest, be encouraged to challenge and deconstruct the frameworks of the subjects they are studying and seek to construct their own.

Connections with existentialism: driving to become an independent thinker

One of the primary goals of problem-based learning is that it intends to help students develop self-directed learning skills. This notion draws from the Existentialist perspective, as articulated by Kierkegaard (1813–55) and Nietzsche (1844–1900), who purported that human existence could be described completely in either scientific or idealistic terms. These philosophers believed that learning should empower a student to become a free, mature and authentic self. Like Aristotle, Kierkegaard believed in the dialectical method and focused on the cognitive and seeing the part within the whole (Malantschuk 1971). Individuals learn by observing others and experimenting rather than being told information (Stendahl 1976). Kierkegaard believed in pursuing given resolutions of problems and arriving either at a verification or rejection of each one. Kierkegaard constructed new viewpoints to establish correctness and places subjects into the new context (Malantschuk 1971). Similarly, Nietzsche believed in learning to think and criticized schools and universities for no longer having any idea about this. Nietzsche questioned the value of educators, as he believed that no one could educate anyone else, that education must necessarily be self-education. Otherwise, education becomes a form of control and levelling. In addition, he believed that students must eventually become teachers themselves. In problem-based learning, students must think for themselves, and take both ownership of their learning and responsibility for teaching peers in their teams.

Connections with postmodernism: the individual and society

Problem-based learning would appear to be an effective pedagogy for women and minority groups since it does not exclude participants in ways that more traditional pedagogies do. This concept has proved essential in the latter half of the twentieth century, when postmodern theories of knowledge have abounded. Modernity was seen as a distinct period of historical development whose origins were in the Enlightenment of the late eighteenth century, which precipitated industrial capitalism and the nation-state. The breakdown of modernity has been seen by many as resulting in the emergence of postmodernism where fragmentation and ambiguity abound. What took place was an epochal shift or break involving the emergence of a new social totality with its own distinct organizing principles. The postmodern world has replaced the modern centres of production such as factories and manufacturing businesses. Instead we have centres of consumption such as theme parks, shopping malls and financial services. Within this consumer society we have lost the production-orientated identity, faith in rationality and science and the notion of progress as human betterment. Instead we see that the fractures of modernity are acknowledged in a postmodern world. Stability, production, clear norms and values are no longer out there. Instead people make their way in a rapidly changing world, where knowledge is constantly on the move and there are few, if any, traditional anchoring points or fixed references. Perhaps the most influential postmodernists are Derrida, Foucault, Lyotard, Irigaray and Cixous. The ideas of these thinkers vary radically, but they do share some common thoughts about knowledge and education, which are characterized by fragmentation and ambiguity, the disintegration of the 'grand narratives' and the challenge to previous conceived notions of objective reality and truth. The postmodernist believes that a person's race, class and gender reflect that person's outlook and although identities are shaped by particular histories, cultures and social relations they are not fixed entities. The self is thus dethroned from its position of agency, freedom and self-determination, and in its place is a panoply of perspectives that acknowledge divergent realities and pluralistic values. Postmodernists are also critical of the society that marginalizes people because of differences and they vigorously defend values of social justice and democracy.

The postmodernists view education as moving beyond knowledge production toward the production of political agents, who will have autonomy and exercise control especially over the conditions of knowledge production and acquisition. Thus the tutor's role is that of a 'transformative intellectual who is engaged in the production of ideologies and social practices' (Giroux 1999: 695). Teachers should assume the stance of social critics who address the political issues of their neighbourhood, nation and wider global world. In the post-modern perspective, tutors are not authoritative experts; rather they participate in inquiry. In a problem-based learning course, tutors and students are often viewed as co-learners so that there is a shift away from staff being the patrollers and controllers of knowledge. Drawing from each of these theoretical underpinnings and occurring at a critical juncture in higher education, marked by increased calls for accountability and change, we share the belief that problem-based learning has developed at an essential time in the evolution of teaching and learning in academe.

Educational origins: medical schools and catalysts for change

As these epistemological notions converged, in Canada and the USA, the twentieth century found higher education and particularly medical education ready for reform. One of the problems lay in the large number of poorly run and privately funded medical schools producing an over-abundant number of physicians in the USA (Flexner 1910). Concerned about the lack of quality, the Carnegie Commission requested Flexner to conduct a comprehensive examination of American and Canadian medical schools. Flexner, perhaps using Johns Hopkins Medical School as his model, argued strongly that medical education should be taken out of the hands of physicians and placed in line with university education, consisting of academic training and clinical practice, linked closely with the science fields. He argued that as they existed, teaching practices were antiquated and dogmatic and instead should encourage students to engage actively in learning and continue to do so over their lifetimes. This report, and a flurry of others, cast a pall over medical education and led to demands for increased accountability. Much of what Flexner suggested was heeded, and as proprietary schools began to close, medical education moved under the domain of academe and began to be linked with academics and clinical practice.

The latter half of the century found medical education at another critical crossroads as it faced growing problems: the information explosion, the fragmentation of the curriculum, and the shortage of graduates with adequate problem-solving and critical thinking skills. Medical educators became increasingly concerned that memorizing propositional knowledge was not creating the long-term learning goals they held. Traditional medical curricula were being called into question for not adequately addressing the challenges raised by Flexner (Camp 1996). Studies were showing that student learning in traditional classrooms was not effective, as students largely forgot the content (Levine and Forman 1973). Perhaps worse, studies were finding that traditional education actually impaired students' natural problem-solving skills (Barrows and Bennett 1972).

Early versions of problem-based learning

In 1966, planning began for a new hospital and medical school in Ontario, Canada, affiliated with McMaster University Medical School (Haslett 2001). This provided an opportunity for developing a new approach to medical education. The readiness for change converged with a recognition of the need for a new medical school with no pre-existing curriculum. Donald Woods of McMaster has been credited for coining the term problem-based learning, and McMaster generally is credited with bringing it to the forefront of education.[1] Preceded by years of questioning, critiquing and final planning, the first class, numbering 19 medical students at McMaster, began in 1969. The early efforts of McMaster met with apparent success on the part of tutors and students (Barrows and Tamblyn 1976, 1977; Camp 1996). Early descriptions of the approach by Barrows and Tamblyn, two educators often credited with the creation of problem-based learning, reveal that McMaster focused on simulating patient problems in a manner consistent with a practising physician. Students worked in small teams and did not receive traditional lectures; instead they used a 'problem pack', which they received in a card deck format (Barrows and Tamblyn 1977). When compared with a control group, students who worked in the problem-based learning format were seen to have increased motivation, problem-solving and self-study skills (Barrows and Tamblyn 1976).

The next decade saw growing interest in this new method, popularized perhaps as a result of Barrows and Tamblyn's research into the reasoning abilities of the McMaster students, which gained ascendance during the 1980s. The research stemmed from a desire to develop in medical students the ability to relate the knowledge they had learned to the problems with which the patients presented, something they found that few medical students could do well. Barrows and Tamblyn's studies highlighted clear differences between problem solving and problem-based learning.[2] Perhaps seemingly contrary to such success, in 1983, McMaster experienced a change in their curriculum. McMaster presented this change, however, as a positive readjustment in their efforts to adapt to the needs of the learner and the proposed learning outcomes of the curriculum. Changes were undertaken to incorporate new knowledge of biology, healthcare and health determinants, to define programme objectives more clearly to improve evaluation processes, and to provide students with more flexibility.

Soon after McMaster began its problem-based learning curriculum, two other new medical schools, at the University of Limburg at Maastricht in the Netherlands and at the University of Newcastle in Australia, adapted the McMaster model of problem-based learning and in so doing developed their own spheres of influence. The University of Limburg (now Maastricht), began a new medical school in 1975, which saw problem-based learning as the primary strategy for the first four study years. The institution developed a new library consistent with the problem-based learning approach in 1992 (Ebenezer 1993). The approach also become popular in Australia, perhaps spurred in part by the Karmel Report in 1973 that concluded that Australian medical school curricula were too science-oriented (Report on the Committee for Medical Schools 1973). The report chastised institutions for staid practices and for neglecting primary care. While this report spurred on change in existing medical schools, it also led to the establishment of a new medical school in Newcastle in 1978, with a mandate for innovative approaches to medical education (Clarke 1978); with this mandate, the institution adopted the problem-based learning model.

In addition to influencing medical education worldwide, McMaster, Maastricht and Newcastle had considerable influence upon each other as well. According to Barrows (2000), many of the educators at Maastricht and Newcastle spent months to years at McMaster while working to develop their new curricula. Fertilization and cross-pollination of ideas allowed the model to grow and also kept the three universities fairly congruent in their approaches. However, there have also been differences in the way in which problem-based learning has been adopted in different disciplines within the institutions,[3] which is something we explore later in this chapter and again in subsequent chapters.

Despite the initial success reported by McMaster, Limburg and Newcastle, not all schools bought into the McMaster model wholesale. Circumstances were different as many had existing curricula that they had to adapt, and curricular change was often difficult. In addition, with existing tutors, staff and administrators, making such a change would require skilfully negotiating complex personality, political and ideological differences. Furthermore, as early as it was in the development of the method, there were few results that indicated its success in the long term. In the face of these and other issues, rather than adopting a traditional McMaster model, many institutions adapted the model to their particular circumstances.

Some institutions developed separate curricular tracks that resembled the McMaster model but ran parallel with their traditional medical school curriculum. The University of New Mexico School of Medicine, which began its problem-based approach in 1979 (Donner and Bickley 1993), stands as a prime example. This university perhaps marked the first break from the McMaster model, as their curriculum educated small numbers of medical students to provide rural, primary care (Barrows 2000). Southern Illinois University's School of Medicine, USA, began its problem-based learning journey when it appointed Howard Barrows as Associate Dean for Educational Affairs in 1981. Barrows has had a significant influence on SIU medical school and the physician's assistant programme. The institution initiated a separate track in 1990 (Allen and Coulson 2000). In this track, a small number of students took the first two years of study (to rejoin the other students in the third year) in a problem-based format that involved tutorial teams of 5–7 students and a tutor. Students did not attend lectures but rather received a set of problems, in either printed form or through standardized patients that were designed for students to learn the content and skills needed from the first two years. Students' tasks involved determining the patient's current condition, taking a medical history, performing a physical examination, ordering diagnostic tests and making an initial hypothesis about the cause of the patient's problem. Southern Illinois University began this track with the goal of moving its entire curriculum to problem-based learning.

Other medical schools, such as Harvard, USA, developed an approach in which students took a certain number of traditional lecture courses interspersed with problem-based learning courses. Implemented in 1985, this curriculum integrated basic science and clinical medicine throughout the entire four years. Students worked with a generalist medical tutor, who stayed with them in the same problem-based learning group throughout their studies. From the initial efforts by McMaster, Maastricht and Newcastle, problem-based learning began to spread (Savery and Duffy 1994). Since its inception, it has been used in European, North American, South American, African and Asian medical schools, including those in the UK, Sweden, Switzerland, Brazil, Chile, South Africa and Hong Kong. With their focus on the whole student as learner, from these three institutions came 'one of the more important educational movements of this century' (Camp 1996).

The professions

As a natural progression from the medical school arena, other health-related programmes began to use problem-based learning from the 1980s onwards. These included programmes such as veterinary medicine at Mississippi State University, USA, pharmacy at Samford University, USA, and nursing at the universities of North Carolina, USA, and Newcastle, Australia. In the UK during the 1980s problem-based learning was adopted in occupational therapy at the then West London Institute of Higher Education and The London Hospital Medical School, and in social work education at the University of Bristol.

Problem-based learning soon began to move beyond its origins in medical schools and the health professions. The use of problem-based learning as a pedagogical approach thus spread from its original inception in medical education and other health-related fields to other professional preparation programmes (Bridges and Hallinger 1996; Casey and Howson 1993; Major 1999) that had similar concerns. Lecturers responded positively to findings from medical-school research such as increased tutor and student satisfaction and increased retention. Problem-based learning was seen as a suitable strategy for professions that were attempting to produce competent practitioners, and problem-based learning soon found a place in several professional schools such as engineering at McMaster and in the UK at Coventry University and Imperial College, London; business at Maastricht, and education at Stanford University, USA. Other disciplines in which problem-based learning is used around the world include architecture, economics, educational administration, law, forestry, optometry, political science and social work (Bridges and Hallinger 1996; Cordeiro and Campbell 1996; Boud and Feletti 1997). Problem-based learning in education for the professions has also been adopted at universities in Denmark, Finland, France, South Africa and Sweden, to name but a few.

Arts, humanities and sciences

We have seen some movement of problem-based learning courses into traditional arts curricula, as tutors and students in these areas have grappled with questions of usefulness and application of these disciplines and as they have struggled for continuation and survival in an era that tends to increasingly value the professions. The spread has occurred as a natural extension of the professions, moving first into the area of science courses. One of the major efforts in arts and sciences occurred at the University of Delaware, USA. Their problem-based learning began as a grassroots movement in the sciences faculty, spearheaded by Duch in the early 1990s. By 1998, the efforts of Duch and colleagues at the University of Delaware were applauded in the Boyer Report (1998), a report from the Carnegie Foundation for the Advancement of Teaching.

Samford University in Birmingham, Alabama began to experiment with problem-based learning across its general and liberal education curriculum in the late 1990s. After the method had gained some ground in both the pharmacy school and the school of education, the Pew Charitable Trusts funded a three-year effort to integrate problem-based learning throughout Samford's undergraduate curriculum, focusing specifically on the areas of general and liberal education. Five schools were involved in this campus-wide effort: arts and sciences, business, education, nursing and pharmacy. The institution hosted an international conference in 2000. It was subsequently awarded a follow-up grant from Pew to encourage tutors to document problem-based learning effectiveness through authentic means such as course portfolios.

Arts and humanities have begun to face questions about their relevance and value in an increasingly market-driven economy which has vast influence on academe, marked by the rapid growth and expansion of professional fields. The increased use of problem-based learning has arguably been slower in these areas, perhaps because of the challenges of adapting the classical model to these subjects. Certainly Hutchings and O'Rourke's work in the UK (Hutchings and O'Rourke 2004) has suggested that 'literary studies is essentially a discursive, open-ended, critically contested, responsive and creative subject that challenges students and encourages them to find their own intellectual pathways'. In their study of problem-based learning in literary studies, Hutchings and O'Rourke found that any imposition of a rigid structure in terms of specific responsibilities within the groups was counter-productive to the nature of learning within the discipline.

Three institutions are notable for 'across the curriculum problem-based learning' extending into the areas of arts and humanities: firstly, Maastricht, founded in 1976 and built from the ground up on a problem-based model. All of its faculties, including the faculty of arts and cultures rely on problem-based learning methods. Second is Åalborg, Denmark, founded in 1974. Åalborg is problem-oriented and project-based, which many distinguish from the problem-based approach. Third is Samford, with perhaps its most unique feature being its efforts to adopt a problem-based model for humanities. Samford and Maastricht have received a grant from the Fund for the Improvement of Secondary Education (FIPSE) to form a transatlantic cooperation for problem-based learning in the humanities.

Further and secondary education

Problem-based learning is being used in further education to some degree in the UK, for example at Edge Hill College. However, the greatest area of growth, that crosses the boundaries of further and secondary education, is that being undertaken in the polytechnics in Singapore. One of the most advanced examples of the use of problem-based learning is that being undertaken at the recently formed Republic Polytechnic where students engage with a problem each day and much of the support and feedback occurs online.

In secondary education problem-based learning began to spread in the 1990s; for example, Illinois Mathematics and Science Academy (IMSA), which serves students with talents in mathematics and science, has adopted problem-based learning programmes and curricula. The model IMSA uses is similar to the medical model in secondary school programmes in science and the social sciences (Gallagher and Stepien 1996). To advance IMSA's mission, the Academy established the Centre for Problem-Based Learning in 1992 that serves as an educational laboratory to engage in problem-based learning research, information exchange, teacher training and curriculum development, from nursery school up to post-secondary educational settings. There is growing interest in problem-based learning in secondary education in the UK and in other countries, but in reality little reported research to date.

Conclusion

The attractions of problem-based learning and its uptake in the 1970s and 1980s in Canada, Australia and the USA, and in the late 1980s in the UK, seemed to lie not only in its timely emergence in relation to other worldwide changes in higher education, but also because of new debates about higher and professional education. These related to a growing recognition that there needed to be not just a different view of learning and higher education, but also a different view about relationships between industry and education, between learning and society, and between government and universities. Such debates continue.

Worldwide expansion in higher education, with the move towards a mass rather than an elite system and a more diverse student population than in former years has demanded tutors use a broader range of teaching and learning methods than before. Flexible approaches to learning and new and different forms of distance education are just a few of the recent demands diverse students require of the higher education system. Such demands have caused many departments to consider using approaches such as problem-based learning to take account of students' requirements. The growth and change has been diverse and varied, spurred forward by individuals, institutions and foundations, and involving a move towards increasing flexibility and adaptability. The growth has also been spurred on by the development of understanding in how people learn, which is the topic of our next chapter.

Notes

1   There is minor debate about where formal problem-based learning first originated. It may have originated at Case Western Reserve University Medical School (USA), when in the late 1950s, the institution incorporated instructional methods and strategies into a multidisciplinary laboratory. In addition, Michigan State University developed a curriculum based around 'focal problems' before problem-based learning emerged, but it did not catch on either.

2   In the former (problem-solving), individual students answered a series of questions from information supplied by a lecturer. In the latter (problem-based learning), students in small teams explored a problem situation and through this exploration examined gaps in their own knowledge and skills in order to decide what information they needed to acquire in order to resolve or manage the situation with which they were presented.

3   These variations have led to interesting attempts to classify what is 'pure' problem-based learning and what is not. We argue that this attempt to classify is prescriptive in nature and does a disservice to the range of forms of problem-based learning currently in use around the world. We argue for a more analytical approach to depicting problem-based learning and outline a variety of models of problem-based learning in Chapter 3.

3

Problem-based learning and theories of learning

Introduction

Problem-based learning emerged from a rich pool of inquiry in how people acquire and transfer knowledge. Ideas that preceded our time have left us with a legacy that underpins current problem-based approaches to teaching and learning. As the field of psychology has gained prominence, the evolving and continuing debates prompted by proponents of different theories about the nature and process of learning have created a minefield of overlapping concepts, with few clear frameworks for understanding the relationship between the context and the experience of the learner. In order to come to terms with these differences, learning theories have traditionally been grouped into categories, the primary ones including behavioural and cognitive theorists, with a range falling somewhere in between, and with full acknowledgement that categories may overlap each other.

While this chapter is by no means an exhaustive account of the psychological or educational perspectives that have influenced the development of problem-based learning, we believe it useful to discuss some of the theories of learning related to the approach. Thus we explore the relationship between problem-based learning and a number of learning theories, namely behavioural, cognitive, developmental and humanistic approaches. Theories of learning that centre on the experience of students and the role of tutors have grown in importance since the 1980s, and therefore we also present theories that focus on the value of meaning construction, personal transition, the learning context and learner identity.

Problem-based learning and behavioural theories

While some behavioural theories seem to run contrary to problem-based learning, the approach has certain elements that can be classified as behavioural in nature, as they gave us some of our first conceptions of how people learn. Some behavioural theories, such as the classical conditioning model posed by Watson and operant condition proposed by Skinner, seem to run contrary to problem-based learning, but theories such as those espoused by Thorndike provided an understanding of improvement of learning through feedback, clear goals and practice, concepts that underpin many forms of problem-based learning. In addition, Hull's work and his notion of Drive Reduction Theory, which asserts that behaviour is determined in part by learner motivation, promotes a key aspect of problem-based learning, which asserts that students should be motivated as stakeholders attempting to solve an important problem.

One of the problems with behavioural notions is that they generally assert that we cannot observe learning except through behavioural changes. Thus they see learning as a relatively permanent change in behaviour brought about as a result of experience or practice. This makes the product or outcome the most important factor, rather than the iterative process of learning that problem-based learning tries to promote. There are other assumptions that emerge from the behavioural tradition as well, such as the belief that outcomes and benchmarking standards will somehow make learning better, or will prove competence to practice, or even make what is taught auditable across the same subject in different universities.

Early behavioural theories took too simplistic a view of learning and have resulted in some lasting influences, such as the development of use of performance objectives in learning. These behavioural objectives are usually manifest in programmed instruction, competency-based education and skill development and training, that are not suitable for understanding the complex learning that we seek in academe, such as learning multifaceted ideas and theories, and developing metacognitive skills. For behaviourists, learning activities should be organized to optimize acquisition of information and routine skill, which is too confining for both problem-based learning and many tutors in higher education.

Problem-based learning and cognitive theories

Unlike behavioural theories, cognitive theories focus on mental processes and thus provide an interesting lens for understanding the origins of problem-based learning. In contrast to the behaviourist theories, cognitive theories are directly concerned with mental processes (which include insight, information processing, memory and perception) rather than products (behaviour), which some would suggest is more in keeping with the process approach of problem-based learning. Cognitive theorists seek to understand how individuals learn and what goes on inside the mind when learning occurs. This kind of education focuses on cognitive structuring which is essential for developing capacity and skills for better learning, or to learn how to learn, one of the primary goals of problem-based learning.

Cognitive theories tend toward the more abstract, as they are generally more difficult to measure or evaluate scientifically than behaviourist theories, much like outcomes in problem-based learning may be more challenging to measure than is performing a specific task taught through skills-based instruction.

Promoters of the cognitive tradition, including Tolman, Koffka, Kohler, Lewin, Piaget, Ausubel and Bruner, have argued that new information has to be interpreted in terms of both prior knowledge and shared perspectives. Thus the existing cognitive structure is the principal factor influencing meaningful learning. In practice this indicates that meaningful material can only be learned in relation to a previously learned background of relevant concepts. Problem-based learning advocates, as well as advocates of other forms of active learning, argue that students enter any learning environment with pre-existing knowledge and cognitive structuring. The focus in this approach thus centres on helping students to utilize their previous knowledge and ways of thinking, and constructing it into a new form that is understandable and meaningful to them.

Maps, gaps and interaction

One of the earliest cognitive theories, bridging the gap from behaviourism to constructivism, came through Tolman's work on sign theory and cognitive mapping. Tolman (1948) believed that learners have goals and follow signs on the way to the goal. Meaningful new stimuli are associated with those already existing to create a cognitive map. Thus he suggested that we create, add to and modify our maps as we learn. As with the behaviourists, for Tolman learning is always purposive and goal-directed. In contrast, the Gestalt theories posited that learning results from experiencing a perceptual whole rather than individual stimuli and can also result from a discontinuous process, which relates to the holistic view of learning that we have come to understand. The focus of the theory, then, is on the idea of grouping and an emphasis on higher-order thinking skills – those skills that are particularly important in the problem-based learning approach.

Wertheimer was particularly interested in problem solving and suggested that the essential aspect was being able to see the overall process. Thus learners should try to find the overall structure of the problem and then the gaps and incongruities are stimuli for learning. In practice this means that instruction should be based on the organization of learning (Ellis 1938; Wertheimer 1923, 1959), which problem-based learning does through providing a problem without all of the information necessary to solve it. The resulting 'gaps' become learning issues for students, who must explore them in order to make progress towards finding viable solutions to the real world problem situation.

More recently there has been increased understanding of the relationship that exists between social development and problem-based learning.

Social development theory posits that social interaction is essential to learning. Vygotsky (1978) proposed the idea of the Zone of Proximal Development (ZPD), which suggests that learners have limited capabilities for learning beyond their current level. Thus effective learning can be reached by providing sufficient challenge without going beyond the learner's capability. This optimal zone can be extended through guidance and collaboration. Therefore in problem-based learning with an experienced facilitator to guide the process and collaboration with peers, a student's optimal zone is extended, and learning often exceeds what tutors and students originally deemed probable or possible.

Deep and surface approaches

The notion of approaches to learning is rooted in the cognitive tradition, emerging from the work of Marton and Säljö (1976a, 1976b) who distinguished two different approaches to learning: those learners who could concentrate on memorizing (surface approaches to learning) and those who put meaning in their own terms (deep approaches to learning). Entwistle (1981) at the University of Lancaster, UK, extended the work of Marton and Säljö in what are known as the Lancaster studies, which were first undertaken to identify the factors associated with academic success and failure at university. Entwistle then built upon the work on surface and deep approaches to learning as well as the work of Pask (1976), who claimed that there are two general categories of learning strategy that can be identified in cognitive tasks: holists, students who identify the main parameters of a system and then filled in the details, and serialist students, who progressively work through details to build up the complete picture as they go.

Ultimately Entwistle extended the definitions of deep and surface categories and also added a third category: a strategic approach. These three approaches are thus delineated by the following characteristics:

- Deep approach
  Intention to understand
  Vigorous interaction with content
  Relate new ideas to previous knowledge
  Relate concepts to everyday experience
  Relate evidence to conclusions
  Examine the logic of the argument
- Surface approach
  Intention to complete task requirements
  Memorize information needed for assessments
  Failure to distinguish principles for examples
  Treat task as external imposition
  Focus on discrete elements without integration
  Unreflectiveness about purpose or strategies

- Strategic approach
  Intention to obtain highest possible grades
  Organize time and distribute effort to greatest effect
  Ensure conditions and materials for studying are appropriate
  Use previous exam papers to predict questions
  Be alert to cues about marking scheme

These approaches connect well with problem-based learning and students may often begin by engaging with the problem using a surface approach and then as they become more experienced tend to adopt deep or strategic approaches. However, an interesting challenge may occur, for tutors and the team, when students with diverse strategic approaches work together since this is likely to result in conflict among team members.

Cognitive development theories

The developmental theorists offer us models that take account of cognition and development. The teacher's concern here is in enabling students to develop both understandings of the nature of knowledge and ways of handling different conceptions of the world, so that knowledge acquisition is seen as an active process. From this field, a number of innovative studies have arisen. Piaget's Cognitive Development theories (Piaget 1929), for example, rely on the notion of cognitive structures. Like Vygotsky, Piaget believed that the activities learners could complete matched their cognitive stage or readiness. Piaget defined four major stages of development from birth where motor actions are developed (Sensorimotor) through to adolescence where abstractions are understood (Formal operations). Piaget's theory is perhaps one of the first that looked at how learners grow and develop over time and how the actual act and process of learning changes. Later Perry extended this concept in his qualitative study of men at Harvard. He devised nine positions that described how students' conceptions of the nature and origins of knowledge evolved (Perry 1970, 1988). This classic study put issues of learner experience centre stage and argued that students proceed through a sequence of developmental stages. In this description of the attainment of intellectual and emotional maturity, the student moves from an authoritarian, polarized view of the world, through stages of uncertainty and acceptance of uncertainty, to finally an understanding of the implications of managing this uncertainty. The student then accepts the need for orientation by adopting a commitment to values and eventually gains a distinct identity through a thoughtful and constantly developing commitment to a set of values.

Belenky *et al.* (1986), stimulated by Perry's work to explore diverse women's perspectives, identified five categories of 'ways of knowing' and from this drew conclusions about the way women saw truth, knowledge and authority. For example, women began from a position of silence where they saw themselves as mindless, voiceless and subject to the whims of external authority. In later stages women constructed knowledge; the women viewed all knowledge as related to the context in which it occurred, and experienced themselves as creators of knowledge. Similarly Ausubel's assimilation theory of learning (Ausubel *et al.* 1978) posits the idea that better learning occurs if people can find meaning in the learning. Learning occurs when a learner is presented with new information that possesses some external or internal characteristics that enables the learner to associate it with previous learning. This theory shares with the Gestalt theories the idea that learning requires a view of the whole. According to Ausubel, advanced organizers, or a bridge between new material and existing ideas, are instrumental for learning. It is the work of these developmental theorists that seems to offer some of the more tenable models of learning. They are models which, to a degree, acknowledge that what is missing from many curricula is a recognition of the role and relevance of learning from and through experience, which can prompt the shaping and reconstructing of people's lives as learners and teachers.

Problem-based learning draws from all of the cognitive theories: students compare new information to existing cognitive structures, they seek to determine the overall structure of the problem, their learning capabilities may be extended through guidance and collaboration, they learn through progression of experience and they learn best when they can see the meaning in learning. Norman and Schmidt assert that research on memory, mastery, transfer and categorization are important parts of problem-based learning from the cognitive psychologist's view (Norman and Schmidt 1992).

Humanist theories

Humanist theories, including the work of psychologists such as Maslow and Rogers, offer us a further understanding of problem-based learning. Maslow (1968) posited a hierarchy of needs that ranged from essential physiological and safety needs to self-actualization and transcendence. These psychologists see learning as a personal act designed to fulfil potential. Learners, they believe, have both affective and cognitive needs so the goal of learning is to become self-actualized and autonomous, and education should facilitate development of the whole person. Those in the humanistic field contend that significant learning is to be obtained only within situations that are both defined by, and under the control of, the learner (for example, Rogers 1983). Learning involves moving to self-development of a fully functioning person. The prior experience of the learner is acknowledged and it is also recognized that students may be constrained by their own negative experiences of learning. In keeping with this theory, in a problem-based learning environment, the tutor (termed in this tradition facilitator) helps to provide a supportive environment in which learners are enabled to recognize and explore their needs. Learning in problem-based learning, like in the humanist tradition, is seen as involving the whole person, and not just the intellect.

Thus educators in this tradition aim to liberate learners and allow them freedom to learn.

Integrative perspectives on learning

As the twentieth century reached its end, it became less useful to categorize ideas about knowledge as 'philosophical', 'psychological', 'behavioural' or 'cognitive'. Rather, ideas have begun to be drawn from various theories in order to develop more integrative perspectives on learning, and several educational theories have emerged. Problem-based learning to some extent symbolizes an integrative approach to learning, since it draws on a number of learning theories while at the same time acknowledging the importance of learning through experience.

Constructivism

Constructivists believe that knowledge is not an absolute, but is rather constructed by the learner based on previous knowledge and overall views of the world. In its concern with mental processes, constructivism shares some qualities with cognitive theories. Yet, in comparing constructivism with behaviourism and cognitive theories, Cooper suggested:

> The constructivist . . . sees reality as determined by the experiences of the knower. The move from behaviourism through cognitivism to constructivism represents shifts in emphasis away from an external view to an internal view. To the behaviourist, the internal processing is of no interest; to the cognitivist, the internal processing is only of importance to the extent to which it explains how external reality is understood. In contrast, the constructivist views the mind as a builder of symbols – the tools used to represent the knower's reality. External phenomena are meaningless except as the mind perceives them . . . Constructivists view reality as personally constructed, and state that personal experiences determine reality, not the other way round.
>
> (Cooper 1993: 16)

Constructivism is a theory that was developed by Bruner along with Tolman, Lewin, Bigge and Allport. Constructivists believe that learners construct knowledge and are predisposed towards learning. They also suggest how knowledge may be structured and sequenced so that it can be learnt, arguing that the learner must be active, because only she can select and interpret information from the environment. Thus constructivism posits that understanding comes from interactions with the environment, cognitive conflict stimulates learning, and knowledge occurs when students negotiate social situations and evaluate individual understanding. Students on problem-based learning courses have the opportunity to construct knowledge for themselves, to make comparisons with other students' knowledge and to refine knowledge as they gain experience (Camp 1996).

Information processing

Miller's conception of information processing is another connecting model, although more dated than other integrative models. Other theorists in this area include Miller (1956); Newell, Shaw and Simon (1958); Gagne and Dick (1983); Anderson (1984) and Rothkopf (1970). According to information-processing models, memory may be episodic, involving recall of events in detail and sequence, or it may be semantic, involving encoding, storage and retrieval of information. The most widely accepted information processing model has three stages:

1   input or sensory registry;
2   short-term memory processing and rehearsal;
3   long-term memory storage.

According to information-processing theorists, a number of factors can affect rote learning, such as meaningfulness, placement of an item within a list, practice or rehearsal, transfer or interference of prior learning, organization (chunking or categorizing), encoding, context and mnemonics. Several factors also affect meaningful learning, such as abstraction (getting the gist), perceived importance, schema from previous learning (Gagne and Dick 1983; Anderson 1984), prior knowledge, inference, misconceptions, text organization and mathemagenic effects (coined by Rothkopf 1970), to refer to learner strategies to assist learning, such as taking notes or answering additional questions (see for example, Miller 1956; Hilgard and Bower 1975, and Good and Brophy 1986).

Norman and Schmidt (1992) assert that the information-processing model is limited, but claim that it has three aspects relevant to the assessment of problem-based learning:

1   Activation of prior knowledge facilitates the subsequent processing of new information (such as small-group discussion), because working through a problem without consulting resources is a mechanism to activate prior knowledge.
2   Elaboration of knowledge at the time of learning enhances subsequent retrieval (for example discussion, note-taking, answering questions).
3   Matching context facilitates recall (the context includes all features of the environment, whether relevant or irrelevant).

They also believe that problem-based learning students retain information longer, are better able to identify causal relationship and may be better able to transfer concepts to new problems.

Andragogy

In an early theory of how adults learn, Knowles (1978) argues that culture does not nurture the development of the abilities required for self-direction. He sees this as being problematic because it promotes a gap between the need (organically) and the ability to be self-directed. Thus the model and practices that he proposes are designed to narrow this gap. Knowles (1978) first argued for four key differences:

1   a change in self-concept,
2   experience,
3   readiness to learn, and
4   orientation towards learning.

He later (Knowles *et al.* 1984) added a fifth about motivation and in 1989 a sixth about a 'need to know'.

   The strengths of the ideology of andragogy are in its focus upon the self-directed learner and its emphasis on the place of the self in the learning process. However, Knowles's ideals are not based on extensive research findings, nor are they a total picture of adult learning. Jarvis (1995) argues the following regarding andragogy:

• it is not a psychological analysis of the learning process,
• it does not describe why specific aspects of experience are relevant,
• it does not generate a learning sequence for an adult.

Experiential learning

A close connection with problem-based learning may be found in the pragmatic work of Dewey (1938), who emphasized the human capacity to reconstruct experience and thus make meaning of it. Dewey believed in education as a process of continuous reconstruction and growth of experience. He believed that the role of the teacher was to organize learning activities that built on the previous experiences of the students and directed them to new experiences that furthered their growth, and that the curriculum should be closely tied to the students' experiences, developmentally appropriate and structured in ways that foster continuity. Dewey opposed theories of knowledge that considered knowledge specialized and independent of its role in problem-solving inquiry. Dewey's work contributed to the concept of active and experiential learning as well as problem-based learning (Fuhrmann 1996), and it has been argued that problem-based learning fits broadly into the experiential learning tradition (Biggs 1999; Savin-Baden 2000).

Transformational learning

Transformational learning is learning that causes change; in particular, transformational learning shapes people in such a profound way that it affects all subsequent learning. Primary contributors to this theory include Mezirow with perspective transformation and transformative learning (Mezirow 1981), Freire with critical pedagogy (Freire 1972, 1974) and Daloz with the developmental character of formal education in adulthood (Merriam 2001). These theories share common assumptions: people having control over their own situations, the capability to reflect upon them and take action to change them; people constructing their own reality to serve different purposes which they validate through interaction and communication with others; and the transformation of individuals resulting in social transformation. For transformative learning to be successful, education must foster a safe, open and trusting environment, much like problem-based learning advocates suggest.

Styles, identity and contexts

The concept of learning styles has suggested that an individual has a consistent approach to organizing information and processing it in the learning environment, yet the model of learning styles developed by Kolb and Fry (1975), in which they suggest there are four learning styles: converger, diverger, assimilator and accommodator is rather too tidy. They argue that a complete learner is someone who has managed to integrate bipolar components of the four learning styles. Although this is a useful model for helping learners to understand something of their approach to learning, it is problematic in that different learning environments demand different learning styles and thus the complete learner must be someone who can either adapt her style or someone who applies a consistent learning strategy across all environments.

Learner identity expresses the idea that the interaction of learner and learning, in whatever framework, formulates a particular kind of identity. The notion of learner identity encompasses positions that students take up in learning situations, whether consciously or unconsciously. Invariably school leavers attending university have an identity largely formulated through their schooling and arrive at university with a sense of whether they are deemed to be successes or failures by peers and external authorities. These students understand themselves in terms of how they are seen as learners by others. They realize components of their learner identity through the eyes of others, even if they cannot define it for themselves. For more experienced students, learner identity is not related to how they are seen by others but instead through the conditions under which they perceive themselves to be learning. Thus learner identity incorporates not only a sense of how one has come to be a learner in a given context, but also the perceptions about when and how one actually learns. As a result, learner identity also encompasses affective components of learning that often seem to matter little to those in the business of creating learning environments in institutional settings. Issues of trust and fear that emerge through critical reflection such as questioning, reframing assumptions, learning together, sharing and evaluating researched information, undertaking presentations and arguing one's point are rarely acknowledged in learning environments (Brookfield 1994). Still, learner identity is not to be seen as a stable entity but as something people use to make sense of themselves, and the ways in which they learn best in relation to other people and the learning environments in which they are learning.

Bernstein (1992) argues that through experiences as students, individuals within higher education are in the process of identity formation. He suggests that this process may be seen as the construction of pedagogic identities that will change according to the different relationships that occur between society, higher education and knowledge. Pedagogic identities are defined as those that 'arise out of contemporary culture and technological change that emerge from dislocations, moral, cultural, economic and are perceived as the means of regulating and effecting change' (Bernstein 1992: 3). Thus pedagogic identities are characterized by the emphases of the time. For example, in the traditional disciplines of the 1960s, students were inducted into the particular pedagogical customs of those disciplines, whereas pedagogic identities of the 1990s were characterized by a common set of market related, transferable skills. The difference between learner identity and pedagogic identity is that, while pedagogic identities are seen to be those that arise out of contemporary culture and technological change, learner identities emerge from the process through which students seek to transcend subjects and disciplines, and the structures embedded in higher education. Thus in developing their learner identities, some students are enabled to shift beyond frameworks that are imposed by culture, validated through political agenda or supplied by academics. They are facilitated in developing for themselves, possibly through learning such as problem-based learning, the formulation of a learner identity that emerges from challenging the frameworks, rather than having the frameworks and systems imposed upon them.

Learning context

The notion of the learning context has been discussed in a variety of ways by authors who have predominantly been concerned with students' learning experiences. For example, Ramsden (1984, 1992) suggested that a student's perception of the learning context is an integral component of his learning. The learning context is created through students' experiences of the constituents of the programmes on which they are studying, namely teaching methods, assessment mechanisms and the overall design of the curriculum.

Students, Ramsden suggests, respond to the situation they perceive, which may differ from that which has been defined by educators. Yet, however much it is denied, educators tend to think of learning contexts as static environments. Each year the programme or module is on offer, and is usually fairly similar to the one offered the previous year and so students are taught in the same way with the same material. It is as if people, and students in particular, are put into contexts and watched while they move about inside them. Yet learning contexts are transient in nature, and much of the real learning that takes place for students occurs beyond the parameters of the presented material.

Taylor (1986) has argued that since educational programmes are temporary environments, it is important to raise students' awareness of the changing natures of the learning environment, peers, tutors and themselves. Therefore, recognition of students' perceptions of the formal learning context is the key to facilitating students' ability to manage learning effectively. However, we argue that the concept of learning context incorporates more than just the students' experiences of the component's teaching methods, assessment mechanisms and the overall design of the curriculum. Equally, learning context comprises more than that which can be defined according to the situation and perhaps even the disciplinary area of study. Thus the notion of learning context incorporates the interplay of all the values, beliefs, relationships, frameworks and external structures that operate within a given learning environment. Learning context also incorporates the way in which the curriculum is situated within the university and the broader framework of higher education, and thus the way it is situated within such systems and frameworks will affect what it means to be a learner in such a context. Furthermore, the notion of learning context does not only comprise the formal curriculum but also the informal ones – the ones students' create for themselves. This might suggest that the smallest component of any learning context could be said to be the formal curriculum, since the learning context is in reality rarely bounded by formal structures but instead by those who comprise and define it.

Conclusion

There are a variety of perspectives about how people learn and all have limitations, but problem-based learning is an approach to learning that has been constructed from a perspective that considers a whole range of theories. While the originators of this approach were medical educators and not trained psychologists or educators, they were influenced by common conceptions about how people learn. It was the context and culture of the time that led to the creation of this approach, which drew from the ideals of what we have come to know and understand about how people learn. They worked to develop an integrated curriculum and our next chapter examines models of curricular practice.

4

Curricula models

Introduction

In this chapter, we explore the ways in which problem-based learning curricula may be put into practice. There are several blueprints for problem-based learning but relatively little information exists to guide those who want to consider how to use it in terms of actually designing the curriculum in a practical way. Cultural and institutional constraints affect the design of problem-based curricula, as do issues that tend to differ across disciplines, such as the way an essay is constructed or the way that knowledge is seen. However, in this chapter we suggest that eight *modes of curriculum practice* are in operation across the problem-based learning community. We present each of these modes and outline some of the advantages and disadvantages of each. These modes are not meant be an exhaustive list but rather a means of considering what occurs in some programmes as well as the impact of opting for a particular design. Such modes also allow us to point up the pitfalls of opting for those that may disable rather than enable student learning.

What is a problem-based learning curriculum?

One of the main difficulties in helping people to understand the difference between problem-based learning and other similar approaches to learning relates to comprehension of curriculum and indeed what might count as a curriculum. We suggest that although we talk about the notion, and construction, of a curriculum, in many ways we do not *have* a curriculum, since curricula are constructed with and through our students. If we speak of the learning intentions we place in the validated programme document in terms of an abiding concern for the life worlds of the students, then we need to examine the process of meaning construction within our subjects and disciplines and clarify how meanings are embodied in the language used by staff and students. Thus the types of questions we might be asking are, 'What does knowing mean in this context?' or, 'How do we create a curriculum that engages students in construction and development of knowing?' Barnett has argued, 'Interpreted broadly and correctly "curriculum" embraces the students' engagement with the offerings put before them. But a curriculum is, in any case, a statement of what counts as knowledge in several senses . . . The medium *is* the message' (Barnett 1994: 45–6).

Curricula where problem-based learning is central to the learning are in fact largely constructivist in nature because students make decisions about what counts as knowledge and knowing. What is problematic here is how such a constructivist stance can be married with benchmarking statements and the emerging audit culture in higher education. In recent years, we have seen such a significant shift towards accountability and transparency that the focus in many curricula is more upon outcomes and less upon learning. For example, if the assumption is that the students must cover a given amount of knowledge in a given time, the focus of the curriculum is likely to be on knowledge acquisition rather than learning. In a programme that is centred on skills acquisition, the focus will be on the way in which knowledge is necessarily useful for practice.

When adopting problem-based learning, the extent to which the curriculum is designed as a whole entity is an important concern. For example, in the UK, degree courses in health and social care are constructed as integrated modular programmes: they are designed as a whole; whereas a course in history may just be a collection of modules, with little if any integration, that students just take in order to gain a degree. Curriculum design thus impinges upon tutors' and students' roles and responsibilities and the ways in which learning and knowledge are perceived. To date there has been little in-depth discussion about the design of problem-based curricula. Instead the discussions have tended to centre on what counts as problem-based learning, ways of implementing it and types of problem-based learning (for example Boud 1985; Barrows 1986). More recently Conway and Little (2000) have suggested that problem-based learning tends to be utilized as either an instructional strategy or as a curriculum design. Instructional strategy is where problem-based learning is largely seen as another teaching approach that can be mixed in with other approaches. Thus, it tends to be used within a subject or as a component of a programme or module, where other subjects may be delivered through lectures. In an integrated problem-based learning curriculum, there is a sense of problem-based learning being a philosophy of curriculum design that promotes an integrated approach to both curriculum design and learning. Here students encounter one problem at a time and each problem drives the learning.

A number of other discussions have emerged about types of problem-based learning, the most basic being that there are two types: the pure model and the hybrid model. The argument here is that either the whole curriculum is problem-based and is modelled on the McMaster version of problem-based learning, whereby students meet in small teams and do not receive lectures or tutorials; or it is the hybrid model, which is usually defined by the inclusion of fixed resource sessions such as lectures and tutorials which are designed to support students. Lectures may be timetabled in advance or may be requested by the students at various points in the module or programme. The so-called pure model is also often termed the medical school model, and is invariably defined as necessarily having a dedicated facilitator for small teams of students, being student centred and being seen to be a good choice for highly motivated, experienced learners in small cohorts (see for example Duch *et al.* 2001). The difficulty with this notion of there only being two types (a pure model and a hybrid model), is that in reality given the current number of forms of problem-based learning in existence, most models would be classed as being hybrid.

However, we believe that current curricular practice is more complex than this. For example, McInnis (2000) in a study of Australian universities found that 74 per cent of academics claimed to be using problem-based learning in their teaching. This would imply that not only are many academics changing their approaches to teaching, but also that problem-based learning continues to be implemented willy-nilly as an instructional approach rather than being seen as an approach that requires embedding as a curriculum philosophy and design. Thus, we outline eight curricula modes that we see in operation. Although there are many more, these seem to be the most common ones. Whilst we recognize that curricula are varied both across disciplines and cultures in terms of length and design, the curricula are represented as three-year programmes since this length is common to many undergraduate programmes worldwide.

Mode 1: Single module approach

In this approach, problem-based learning is implemented in one module (possibly two) in one year of a programme, invariably the last year. The lecturer who runs the module is interested in improving student learning and improving students' ability to think critically, something she believes they may not have done, or not done enough of elsewhere in the degree.

The module is often designed using the McMaster model, where students engage with one problem at a time and meet two or three times with the tutor over the course of each problem. Supporting lectures may appear infrequently, if ever, but the tutor may act as resource for the team. Students may not have a facilitator allocated to each team; instead the tutor tends to move around the team or allows the students to run the sessions themselves. The module is invariably different from all the others that the students have encountered earlier in the degree; examples can be seen in engineering (Cawley 1997) and English literature (Hutchings and O'Rourke 2002).

Mode 2: Problem-based learning on a shoestring

This type of problem-based learning occurs with minimal cost and interruption to other areas of the programme. It is usually undertaken by a few tutors who are keen to implement it, perhaps in the face of resistance on the part of other tutors; so it is done quietly and cheaply. It is a model that can be seen in many subjects and disciplines and tends to occur where it has been agreed by the head of department that some tutors can use problem-based learning in some areas of the curriculum. The McMaster model serves as a blueprint for implementation, and the modules appear almost in isolation from the rest of the curriculum. It tends to be implemented in modules run by tutors interested in it and avoided by those who disagree with it. The result is that problem-based learning may be used in few or many modules throughout the curriculum (see Table 4.1), but there is little real rationale for its implementation in particular areas. Thus, the problems used tend to be subject- or discipline-based and rarely transcend disciplinary boundaries. The module may have several problems occurring concurrently, and staff may use lectures to guide the learning. In Mode 2, problem-based learning modules tend to be scattered throughout the programme, students may not understand the rationale for its use, and staff implementing it may often feel frustrated by the lack of departmental or institutional support for their problem-based learning on a shoestring.

Table 4.1 Mode 2: Problem-based learning on a shoestring

Year 1	PBL	Lecture-based	Lecture-based	PBL	Lecture-based
Year 2	Lecture-based	PBL	Lecture-based	PBL	Lecture-based
Year 3	Lecture-based	Lecture-based	Lecture-based	PBL	PBL

Mode 3: The funnel approach

In this mode, the decision has been made by the curriculum design team or head of department to design the curriculum in a way that enables students to be funnelled away from a more familiar, lecture-based approach, towards a problem-based learning approach. They commence with lecture-based learning in the first year, then move on to problem-solving learning in their second year and then problem-based learning in their final year. Thus in the first year, students will receive lectures and tutorials and attend tutor-led seminars. The second year will comprise problems that are set within, and bounded by, a discrete subject or disciplinary area. In this year students will be expected to discover the answers expected by the tutor, answers that are rooted in the information supplied to them through lectures, workshops and seminars. The solutions are always linked to specific curricula content, and it is expected that the students would cover this information before they can funnel into the problem-based learning approach in the third year. The third year is designed with a cohesive framework using problems that build upon one another.

Table 4.2 Mode 3: The funnel approach

Year 1	Lecture-based learning
Year 2	Problem-solving learning
Year 3	Problem-based learning

The decision to design the curriculum in such a way has invariably emerged from a number of tutors' concerns that may include the following:

- tutors' beliefs that students need foundational knowledge and principles before they can engage with problem-based learning;
- tutors' own lack of confidence in their ability to facilitate problem-based learning teams; by using problem-solving learning first, they believe that they will develop the capabilities necessary to make them effective facilitators;
- tutors' beliefs that the students, on entry to the programme, are of such diverse capabilities that many of them will require considerable support in learning and that problem-based learning will be an approach that is too difficult for many of them to undertake initially;
- tutors' assumptions that the professional body who validates the programme will be more content with the funnel approach, as problem-based learning is often seen as being a high-risk approach when educating students for the professions;
- tutors' beliefs that problem-solving learning coupled with plenty of guidance will help students not only develop the capabilities for undertaking problem-based learning but also prevent them from struggling with it;
- tutors' feeling that it is necessary to support and take prodigious care of their students.

Mode 4: The foundational approach

The foundational approach is invariably one that is seen in science and engineering curricula. Here it is assumed that some knowledge is necessarily foundational to other knowledge and, therefore, it needs to be taught to the students before they can begin to solve problems. Thus, in the first year of a programme adopting this approach, the focus is on providing students with lectures, tutorial and laboratory time that will enable them to understand the required knowledge and concepts.

In the second and third year, students then utilize problem-based learning. One of the underlying principles of this approach is the assumption that if basic concepts are taught first, then the knowledge will be decontextualized and will, therefore, be available in the students' memories for use in solving new problems. For example, Eva *et al.* (1998) have suggested that the problem-solving theories concerning ways in which students transfer knowledge from one context to another fall into two broad areas:

• abstract induction: which presumes that students learn principles or concepts from exposure to multiple problems by abstracting a general rule, thus it is independent of context;
• conservative induction: which assumes that the rule is not separated from the problem context but that expertise emerges from having the same principle available in multiple problem contexts.

Thus advocates for such programmes take the view that by teaching principles of problems, students will then use these principles to solve other similar problems. Inevitably, this raises questions about the extent to which problem-solving can be classed as a generalizable skill and whether some knowledge is necessarily foundational to other knowledge, but we discuss this further in Chapter 7.

A relevant study was conducted by Kandlbinder and Mauffette (2001), which examined theories of teaching 'basic concepts' in sciences in programmes that used student-based learning approaches, including problem-based learning. They suggested that what many lecturers referred to as basic concepts were in fact far from basic. What emerged from their data were four descriptions of what basic concepts were meant to represent to the students. The metaphor of building was central to the notion of disciplinary understanding, and knowledge was seen as the ability to test propositions rather than the learning of a body of knowledge through rote memorization: 'Basic concepts can also form the boundary of received knowledge, providing identity to the discipline. By their nature these concepts are a particular kind of knowledge that is difficult to locate ... In these cases science university teachers talk about finding the essence of the discipline, particularly in terms of the traditions of science.' (Kandlbinder and Mauffette 2001: 49).

In the foundational approach, the second year generally begins with an introduction to the concept of problem-based learning and possibly some team-building activities. The problems presented to students are ones that demand the use of knowledge and formulae presented to them in the first year. This mode tends to focus on students developing their abilities to resolve and manage problems. Students may be strongly tutor guided in this second year. However, by the third year students are encouraged to take a stance towards knowledge and are often given problems that are from, or relate directly to, industry. (For an example of this type of curriculum see Gibbs 1992: 59–76; Savin-Baden 2000, chapter 3, Lembert University). The difference between the funnel approach and the foundation approach is that in the funnel approach tutors are concerned to guide students towards the problem-based learning process from early on in the curriculum. In the foundation approach tutors believe that some knowledge is necessarily foundational to other knowledge and therefore students must know this foundational knowledge before they can begin to undertake problem-based learning.

Table 4.3 Mode 4: the foundational approach

Year 1	Lecture-based learning
Year 2	Problem-based learning
Year 3	Problem-based learning

Mode 5: The two-strand approach

In the two-strand approach, problem-based learning is seen by tutors as a vital component of the curriculum that has been designed to maximize the use of both problem-based learning and other learning methods simultaneously. This approach also tends to be adopted in universities where tutors might want to implement problem-based learning wholesale across the curriculum but are prevented from doing so because the curriculum is serviced by other disciplines.

Table 4.4 Mode 5: The two-strand approach

Year 1	Problem-based learning modules
	Mixed approach modules
Year 2	Problem-based learning modules
	Mixed approach modules
Year 3	Problem-based learning modules
	Mixed approach modules

For example, in such *serviced modular curricula* (Savin-Baden 2003) what occurs is that a curriculum is designed in, for example, business studies or social work, and both of these curricula require that students study law. However, law is not taught by business studies or social work tutors experienced in business or social work law, but instead their curricula are serviced by academics from the law faculty. Students are thus taught law in a way that is decontextualized from their subject. The information that is taught is rarely applied to practice, and students find it difficult to understand how it is related to other learning that has occurred in different modules. The two-strand approach may also be adopted where there is a university require-ment for students to undertake shared modules across the disciplines, such as research modules, that are not necessarily problem-based.

In the two-strand approach the curriculum has clear strands running alongside one another. The problem-based modules are designed to build on each other but also to draw from the modules in the mixed approach strand. What tends to happen is that modules in each strand are designed with interlocking themes so that the knowledge and capabilities in the mixed approach feed in to support problem-based learning rather than working against it.

Mode 6: Patchwork problem-based learning

The patchwork approach is a complex mode that students often experience as difficult or confusing. Here the whole curriculum is designed using prob-lem-based learning, but due to institutional requirements, the modules do not run consecutively but concurrently. The result may be seen in Table 4.5 where students undertake two or three problems simultaneously in different, but not necessarily related, subject areas. Furthermore, modules are unlikely to last the same length of time, so students may do one problem over a period of four weeks, another over two weeks, and another within a week. Students in this form of curriculum experience problem-based learning as both a disparate and demanding process that tends to result in the com-partmentalization of knowledge, rather than as a means of helping them to integrate it across disciplinary boundaries.

This mode often emerges out of the combination of prescriptive university requirements for curricula to be defined in particular ways, and tutors feel-ing that they need to cover vast amounts of material within particular modules. This mode may also be seen when students, particularly in the USA system, choose to undertake only problem-based learning modules to make up their programme, resulting in a patchwork of knowledge and experience.

Table 4.5 Mode 6: Patchwork problem-based learning

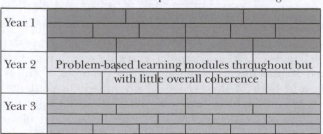

Mode 7: The integrated approach

The integrated approach is based on the principle that problem-based learning is not merely a strategy but a curriculum philosophy. In practice, relatively few examples of this mode of curriculum exist, although it is an approach that many espouse. This model is based on the McMaster model whereby students work in teams, encounter one problem at a time and are facilitated by a tutor. The curriculum exists in an integrated fashion so that all the problems are sequential and are linked both to one another and across disciplinary boundaries. Students are equipped for the programme through explanations of the approach and team-building activities. However, assessments are not necessarily structured to match the aims and values of the curriculum – although this is desirable. For example, in many integrated programmes, multiple-choice questions and examinations may still be used to assess students despite the focus on the process of learning in this mode. Such assessment can thus undermine the student-centred, self-directed focus of this kind of curriculum.

Table 4.6 Mode 7: The integrated approach

Year 1	Problem 1	Problem 2	Problem 3	
Year 2	Problem 4	Problem 5	Problem 6	
Year 3	Problem 7	Problem 8	Problem 9	Problem 10

Mode 8: The complexity model

This mode is an approach to curriculum design that transcends subjects, disciplines and university curriculum impositions, and embraces knowledge, self, actions and curriculum organizing principles. Although Barnett and Coates (2002) have not termed it as such, we would argue here that in their notion of curriculum, what they are proposing is a complexity model, since it reflects the earlier work of Barnett (1997) on supercomplexity. The model takes Barnett's earlier notion of curriculum a stage further and seeks to embed his theorizing in a view of curriculum that reflects the fragmented world of both the learners and the curriculum designers. The model of curriculum proposed by Barnett and Coates is based on an understanding of modern curricula as an educational project forming identities founded in three domains: those of knowledge, action and self. The 'knowledge' domain refers to the discipline-specific competences. The 'action' domain includes those competences acquired through 'doing': such as an oral presentation in art history. The 'self' domain develops an educational identity in relation to the subject areas. What they suggest is that the weight of each of the three domains varies across curricula, and that the domains may be integrated or held separately (but it is not entirely clear how this works), and finally curricular changes tend to be dominated by epistemological differences in the disciplines. What this means in practice is:

> The curricula in science and technology courses are heavily weighted towards the knowledge domain. The domains are held separate (there is little or no integration between the domains). The arts and human-ities curricula are also heavily weighted by the knowledge domain, but here there is more integration with the self domain. In the professional subject areas, there is a high degree of integration across the three domains.
>
> (Barnett and Coates 2002)

In reality this means that the mode of curriculum practice becomes one of problem-based learning for critical contestability (Savin-Baden 2000). What we mean is that problem-based learning of this sort enables students to develop a critical position from which to interpret the practice of others, to (re)develop their own critical perspectives and thence to critique them. This form of problem-based learning is one that seeks to provide for the students a kind of higher education that offers, within the curriculum, multiple models of action, knowledge, reasoning and reflection, along with opportunities for the students to challenge, evaluate and interrogate them. Students will, therefore, examine the underlying structures and belief systems implicit within a discipline or profession itself, in order not only to understand the disciplinary area but also its credence. They will transcend and interrogate disciplinary boundaries through a commitment to exploring the subtext of those disciplines. Knowledge here is seen as being constructed by the students, who begin to see themselves as creators of knowledge, and who become able to build upon and integrate previously learned knowledge and skills with material that is currently being learned. Students are encouraged to evaluate critically both personal knowledge and propositional knowledge on their own terms; thus the student embraces knowledge and also queries it.

As future practitioners it is intended that students would be enabled to become questioning and critical practitioners – practitioners who would not only evaluate themselves and their peers effectively, but would also be able to analyse the shortcomings of policy and practice. Students involved in this form of problem-based learning would tend to adopt reflective pedagogy. They will see learning and epistemology as flexible entities, perceive that there are also other valid ways of seeing things besides their own perspective, and accept that all kinds of knowing can help them to know the world and themselves more effectively. Problem-based learning of this sort enables stu-dents to develop a critical position from which to interpret the practice of others, to (re)develop their own critical perspectives and thence to critique them.

The difficulties with this model largely stem from issues of power and control in the learning context. Tutors' sense of self is likely to feel at risk or threatened in their role in the team and in relation to their conceptions of learning and knowledge, since they will be under increasing scrutiny from the students. It might be that the enactment of this model is only actually possible in the context of postgraduate programmes, where students are offered more freedom to learn in the context of their own agenda than in undergraduate or pre-registration (professional) curricula.

While it would seem to be the model with the best fit for problem-based learning for critical contestability across all disciplines, two important questions are omitted from Barnett and Coates's curriculum framework. The first is the issue of assessment: how do we assess a pedagogy for supercomplexity? The second is how do we manage the relationship between a pedagogy for supercomplexity and competence to practice? In order for this model to work in practice within the context of a problem-based learning curriculum, these questions would need to be addressed. What we suggest is that assessment should enable learning through a reconceptualization of failure as progression and personal development, and that the notion of competence to practice is focused on capabilities for practice. This shifts learning in education for the professions away from a view of student learning as knowledge consumption towards a position of seeing learning as a process of knowledge management.

Conclusion

In problem-based curricula the problem scenarios should serve as the central component of each module so that lectures, seminars or skill laboratories can feed into them in order to inform students, rather than offering them great chunks of propositional knowledge that they may find difficult to integrate into their understanding. Designing a curriculum based on content and disciplinary knowledge and then trying to make it problem-based usually ends in disaster. So whether it is a module or a whole programme that is designed to be problem-based, the starting point should be a set of problem situations that will equip students to become independent inquirers, who see learning and epistemology as flexible entities and perceive that there are also other valid ways of seeing things besides their own perspective. However, it is important to examine the context and culture in which the curriculum is placed, and it is to this that we turn in the next chapter.

5

Cultural contexts of academe

Introduction

Part 1 has examined some of the abstract ideas and theoretical constructs that provide the foundations of problem-based learning. So far in this section, we have delineated the core concepts and have provided information about the philosophical, psychological and educational underpinnings of the method, along with some of the historical origins of problem-based learning. We have also discussed modes of curricular practice. This leads us naturally into the last conceptual frame, which is an examination of academic culture. Understanding the concept of culture and how problem-based learning is situated within its interrelated constructs is essential to understanding the foundational underpinnings of the approach. This section explores conceptions of both culture and academic culture, addresses some of the different dimensions of culture and outlines components of cultural change.

Understanding culture

Culture is an ambiguous term at best, and it has had several different constructs. In attempting to determine what counts as culture many definitions have arisen. One of the pertinent ones is that culture involves the act of developing the intellectual and moral faculties especially by means of education. Another definition indicates that culture is the learned behaviour of a society or group, while a further definition suggests that culture is an integrated pattern of knowledge, belief and behaviour that depends upon human capacity for learning and transmitting knowledge to succeeding generations. It is the customary beliefs, social forms and material traits of a group and the set of shared attitudes, values, goals and practices that characterizes an organization. A formal definition of culture is:

a pattern of shared basic assumptions invented, discovered or developed by a given group as it learns to cope with its problems of external adaptation and internal integration that has worked well enough to be considered valid and therefore, is taught to new members of the group as the correct way to perceive, think and feel in relation to those problems.

(Schein 1985: 9)

Culture, then, acts as a unifying framework that combines the different aspects of life into some kind of whole. Schein suggests that culture may consist of three levels. It consists of basic shared assumptions (including assumptions about the nature of truth), the nature of human activity, and the relationship of the culture to the environment. These views are often unconscious and are invisible to participants in the culture. Culture also consists of shared values, which are more visible to the participants as they often articulate and act on them. Finally, culture consists of creations of the group, which may embody artwork, technology and observable behaviour. Culture may serve four general purposes:

1   it conveys a sense of identity;
2   it facilitates commitment to an entity, such as a university or peer group, other than self;
3   it enhances the stability of a group's social system;
4   it is a sense-making device that guides and shapes behaviour (Kuh and Whitt 1988: 10)

One common trait that these definitions share is the identification of culture as a fixed system. In addition, according to all of the definitions, culture is perpetuated by education and example. Thus, culture by definition is formalized and unchanging and education/socialization of new members is seen as protecting the existing system. In this sense, culture may be seen as divisive if this notion is carried out to the extent that the 'routine' is considered normal and different activities from the routine are considered abnormal (Kuh and Whitt 1988). However, cultures constantly evolve in response to changes in the environment; 'no culture stands still' (Venkatesh 1995: 30) because it is taught and learned, and it changes during migration, conversion and exposure to external and modifying influences. Therefore, culture may be seen as an impeding force of change. It can be what stands in the way of, and even defeats, innovation. However, obstruction and prevention need not be the case as culture will not necessarily have a negative affect on attempted innovation, particularly if culture is understood, and if attempts at change and innovation are appropriately introduced and managed.

The question arises as to how we understand culture, particularly since it is such an ambiguous concept. The study of culture has come into vogue as of late, with little wonder; if culture is such a powerful force, attempts must be made to understand it. It is perhaps because culture itself is such a vague concept that the practice of studying culture has not developed any set structures or methods, and in fact draws freely from a range of disciplines including humanities, social science, science and technology.

Dimensions of academic culture

Academic culture is a specific kind of culture and it is receiving increased attention in the literature of organizational theory and of higher education. Culture in higher education involves 'the collective, mutually shaping patterns of norms, values, practices, beliefs and assumptions that guide the behaviour of individual and groups in an institute of higher education and provide a frame of reference within which to interpret the meaning of events and actions on and off campus' (Kuh and Whitt 1988: 12–13).

Tierney and Rhoads (1994) describe academic culture as the nexus of several forces, of which we will now consider national, disciplinary, subject-specific and institutional culture. Although these are conceptualized as distinct subcultures, these forces are synergistic and do not operate independently of one another.

National culture

Academic culture is situated within the context of national culture and this culture exerts its influence on teaching and learning in academe. Western culture, for example, may be seen as casual and egalitarian (more casual in the USA than in the UK, perhaps) and the focus of the culture is on the individual. Western culture tends to value science and technology. Asian culture, on the other hand, is often seen as polite and formal. In this culture, roles may be prescribed and may involve hierarchy and subordination. It is often seen as a collective culture, in which the needs of the group outweigh the needs of the individual. In contrast, Hispanic culture seems religiously-oriented. Here there is an intersection of the physical and religious world. While these examples may be viewed as stereotypes, we include them to illustrate how, nationally, culture can have a fundamental influence on teaching and learning. In a more traditional culture that values strict lines of authority, for example, problem-based learning may be more of a revolutionary change as tutors and students have an equal footing with one another. In more individualistic cultures the idea of collaborating with peers may be a greater challenge than in more collective ones.

Disciplinary culture

Disciplinary culture exerts a strong influence on academe as it is organized by conceptions of knowledge. Curricula are established on existing understanding about the nature of knowledge and how it should be organized.

Such cultures also have established norms and modes of inquiry as well as values and ways of thinking and feeling. While new interdisciplinary views are taking traditional structures to task and are creating new interdisciplinary programmes of study, many traditional disciplines are still found on college campuses, whether they are English, mathematics, biology or physics.

However, disciplinary culture influences institutions by the very kinds of disciplines that are included on a campus. Campuses may even be categorized by the kinds of disciplines that are present: traditional arts schools, which still focus heavily on traditional humanities, comprehensive universities, which provide a variety of disciplines including some of the more practical professions, or research institutions, which may include some of the more highly technical or professional subjects, such as medicine or engineering. This kind of culture also heavily influences tutors. It is suggested that some tutors have even stronger allegiances to their disciplines than they have to their institutions and to other tutors on campus. This is in part because of the professionalization of tutors, who have become so specialized in their fields that they may well have more in common with their counterparts in other countries than with individuals on their home turfs. Humanities culture, for example, is quite different from physics culture and tutors and students socialized into these different fields have different values, attitudes and preferences. In addition, the relationship is reciprocal, as tutors with certain learning and teaching styles may drift naturally towards specific disciplines.

Disciplinary culture also influences students who select certain tracks or paths within particular disciplines. They, like tutors, may tend to drift toward particular fields because of interest or preference. In addition, though, disciplinary modes of discourse can have great influence on student development, as they establish professional identities congruent with their fields. The ever-expanding role of research has also changed disciplinary culture, along with increasing demands by government for socially relevant research.

Culture affects teaching practices, and thus learning and assessment differ depending upon the nature of the discipline. For example, mathematics and other related subjects tend to focus on general problem solving and the need for correct solutions. At first glance it may seem that a shift to problem-based learning will not be difficult. However, Bowe and Cowan (2004) have reported that the shift from problem solving to problem-based learning in physics was a complex disciplinary shift for both tutors and students. In addition, in the professions, it is easy to picture what kind of problem a professional might face, so it is not a huge leap to develop a problem. In literary studies, collaborative learning may be fairly common, so the shift to using problem-based learning is often easier, but the models of group work and problems management suggested by proponents such as Barrows and Tamblyn (1980) may also seem too restricting for those accustomed to flexible learning patterns where critique is central to disciplinary learning.

Institutional culture

The notion of institutional culture is beginning to receive some attention. Tierney and Rhoads have argued that a state and its organizations tend to exist as social constructions since they revolve around shared understandings. This form of organizational culture shapes behaviour and expectations and academe, as a kind of organization, falls within this definition. Some of the variables that affect institutional culture include type, mission, size, location and character (for example, public or private universities in the USA, and pre- and post-1992 universities (old and new, in the UK).

Thus elite institutions have vastly different cultures to those that value access and opportunity for all. If an institution is dedicated to providing a liberal education, it may have a vastly different culture from one that is attempting to provide students with a more professional or vocational education. A religious institution will have a different culture from a secular one. Some institutions may value traditions, while others value progressive ideals and innovations. Small institutions are likely to have different cultures to large ones, with the small institution perhaps being more cohesive than the large multiversity. Although some writers have tried to outline characteristics of positive campus culture, there is no one correct kind of institutional culture, as institutions are quite diverse, despite what government policies, initiatives and rewards would lead us to believe. Institutional differences in goals, objectives, values and missions may have a direct influence on how innovation is perceived and accommodated, how much change of different kinds can be accomplished and what support is received from government.

In many countries governments want to exert increasing control on universities by rewarding particular forms of research and teaching and exerting pressure through stringent regulatory mechanisms. Thus if, as Ashworth (2003) has suggested, one built a 'meme' – a cultural element comparable with a gene, it could be used as a performance indicator for universities. Dawkins (1990), who coined the word meme in his book *The Selfish Gene* defines it simply as a unit of intellectual or cultural information that survives long enough to be recognized as such and which can pass from mind to mind. Individual slogans, catchphrases, melodies, icons, inventions and fashions are typical memes. An idea or information pattern is not a meme until it causes someone to replicate it, to repeat it to someone else. Memes should be regarded as living structures, not just metaphorically but technically.

The meme that Ashworth builds is a performance indicator for universities. The criteria for such a meme (performance indicators) are excellence in research, teaching and widening participation. Ashworth analysed the ratings that UK universities received in these three categories and found that 38 UK universities had high ratings for teaching and research, 8 universities had high research and participation ratings and 8 universities had high teaching and participation ratings. However, only 2 universities had high research and teaching, and a relatively high proportion of working-class students – Brunel University and Queen's University, Belfast. Thus the hostile environment and anomalous government initiatives that expect all UK universities to be proficient in all three categories will mean that hostile selection is likely to lead to the ultimate extinction of those with low ratings in at least one category. The particular selection pressures evident on universities Ashworth suggests are:

- Economics of the university – does it pay?
- Quality assurance – does it show research-based teaching decisions?
- Technical rationality – does it work?
- Elitism – which universities do it most?
- The relationship between discipline-specific pedagogies as opposed to generic ones.
- Counter claims of other research demands.
- Criteria for research assessment.

We would argue that the naive expectations held by governments that adopt such rating scales and the rewards systems used by such governments around the world, are resulting in an over-compliant university culture that is performative and that is not doing its job in terms of fulfilling the underpinning reasons for being a university. Perhaps the question we need to be asking is not, 'What is a university doing?' but 'What is a university for?' Is there space in the marketplace to manage diverse university cultures which take account of different students, disciplines, teaching approaches and research, whether blue skies or socially responsive? Or as Barnett (2003) has asked, 'Is a university possible?' However, he does give us hope: 'Universities are not, in the first place, sites of knowing but of being. The knowing comes, if at all, through the being. Commitment to hard sustained work calling for critical engagement with others – whether in teaching, research or consultancy – requires a sense of well-being' (Barnett 2003: 179).

Perhaps we should see the university not as a meme in the negative sense, but rather as a positive meme that shifts and changes to reflect the culture of its time, and as a place for challenging policies, practices and thinking systems. The university should be seen as a living structure, a place of being for its tutors and students, with a variety of interrelated memes with different types of energy and opportunities.

Accomplishing innovation and change within pre-existing cultural contexts

Despite the many claims that the paradigm has shifted in higher education from a traditional instructional paradigm to a learning paradigm (McDaniel 1994; Barr and Tagg 1995; Cambridge 1996; Fischetti *et al.* 1996; Farmer 1999), planning for widespread change within a bounded cultural context (such as within an institution of higher education) is still a challenging task. Barriers and resistance to change are common. In particular, pre-existing long-held institutional values, beliefs and norms can impede change efforts. Tierney and Rhoads define socialization as 'the process through which individuals acquire the values, attitudes, norms, knowledge and skills needed to exist in a given society' (Tierney and Rhoads 1994: 6). They argue that socialization occurs in two overlapping stages: anticipatory socialization and organizational socialization. The anticipatory stage relates to how non-members adopt the actions and values of the group to which they aspire. The organizational stage, on the other hand, involves initial entry and role continuance. Noting the importance of the transition process, Tierney and Rhoads comment that when anticipatory socialization and organizational socialization are consistent then the socialization process is affirming. When socialization experiences are inconsistent, the organization will attempt to modify or transform the reality for members of a given culture. While speaking specifically of tutor socialization, their definition aptly situates culture as a process of transmission and as the creation of a professional identity. This definition has applications for administrators, tutors and students as they prepare for instructional change to an existing cultural context. As a result of deeply embedded and shared values, beliefs and norms, organizational culture may play a more significant role in universities than in other types of institution. Therefore, understanding cultural forces can help leaders to interpret stakeholders' visions and thus shape the ways that change can occur. For example, on a university campus, tutors can generate and often sustain culture, and administrative leaders may use that culture to strengthen the organization. In addition, students can exert tremendous power to influence culture, and to bring about the innovations they believe will have to succeed for effective change to occur, which in several universities has resulted in an increase in demand by students for problem-based learning.

Unfortunately, academic institutions often lack the structures necessary to nurture unifying aspects of culture, and to allow change within an existing system. The use of appropriate structures and strategies targeted at supporting and changing culture represents a potentially powerful means of managing change in academic organizations. By working *with* staff who want to develop ideas and promote innovation it is possible to enable change both within departments and across an institution.

Leadership for change

Change can be encouraged at many levels from policy makers to students. Each can exert influence on change at various levels and times, and each have various structures for change at their disposal. However, we argue that effective leadership is essential for establishing change on campus. Leadership can help establish departmental educational goals for teaching and research, and provide vision for change as well as support for tutors and students attempting to effect change. Leaders, whether they are tutors, students or administrative staff, can create, embody, change or integrate cultures at their institutions. Maxwell (1998) has suggested that there are 21 indispensable qualities of a leader that range from character to vision, whereas Fisher (1999) suggests that we just need two! He suggests that leaders need to be visionaries and masters of change. There have however been some less prescriptive texts that take into account the complexities of people and their lives and that offer helpful insights about what it might mean to be a leader. For example, Davison and Ward (1999) suggested that what is appropriate, and when, depends on the cultural context, arguing:

> So if participative leadership means allowing people to speak as and when they want to, then the Australians were more participative than Hong Kong Chinese. If, however, participative leadership means stimulating open-ended unbiased consultation and allowing direct statements of disagreement and criticism, then Hong Kong Chinese were more participative than Australians.
>
> (Davison and Ward 1999: 51–2)

We suggest that what seems to be more relevant is not the particular characteristics of leaders and leadership but the culture and context in which the leadership is taking place. Thus, we would further suggest that university leadership should be of a type that can encompass many situations, suit many styles, and is capable of being embraced by all: *meta-leadership*. Meta-leadership is characterized by a focus on the possibilities. It is future thinking; possibility thinking and creative thinking, thinking that takes us beyond the constraints of our present and allows us to consider the possibilities open to us. Meta-leadership questions the current assumptions, challenges the traditions and breaks self-imposed constraints of caution and conservatism. As such, meta-leadership asks that we risk the anathema of thinking that we may be wrong in our current understanding and, therefore, limited in our current view of the possibilities. Such meta-leadership is vital for the promotion of problem-based learning as an institutional strategy, as it depends upon seeing supercomplexity as an organizing principle of institutional culture. Leaders therefore need to:

- *Challenge common conceptions of teaching.* Tutors and leaders will need to work together to articulate and agree on the meaning of the scholarship of teaching and on what counts as effective teaching.
- *Develop strong advocates.* One of the most important areas that can promote change is letting strong voices be heard. Individuals can commit to, and lead educational innovation, and serve as an advocate for educational reform to tutors, the administration, professional organizations and the general public. Individuals, whether tutors or students, can also advocate grassroots change.
- *Promote cross-campus collaboration.* One of the difficulties with a strong disciplinary culture is that tutors, particularly at larger institutions, rarely interact with those outside their immediate areas, in particular on issues

related to teaching and learning. Interaction among departments on campus can foster an understanding of how particular courses fit the needs of students in other curricula and it can provide ideas that might not otherwise emerge. This kind of support can provide tutors with opportunities and autonomy to experiment, as well as providing the security in which experimentation can thrive.

• *Facilitate the acquisition of resources and funding.* One of the greatest avenues for wielding change is through the provision of financial support. Funding can take the form of direct grants for instructional activities, or be given to individual tutors, departments or institutions. However, reduced resources and funding in higher education in the late 1990s and early 2000s has been problematic in all programmes, whether they use problem-based learning or not. This is due, in the main, to teaching larger numbers with the same or fewer resources. Drinan (1991) argued that constant awareness of the use and purposes of problem-based learning across the curriculum could lead to problem-based learning curricula being no more expensive than traditional ones. Yet there is still much controversy, particularly with regard to library costs, classroom allocation and tutor support for problem-based learning. However, Mennin and Martinez-Burrola (1990) studied the cost of problem-based learning compared with conventional curricula and demonstrated only very small differences. They also found that in problem-based learning curricula 70 per cent of tutor time was in contact with students, while on conventional courses 70 per cent of tutor time was in preparation for contact with students. From this it would seem that funding comparisons between problem-based learning courses and other courses might just be a question of emphasis.

• *Provide and promote academic development.* The increase in the use of problem-based learning has brought with it a great demand for tutor and educational development. In some disciplines and countries the focus is on tutor development; in others, it is on educational development (an area we discuss further in Chapter 10). However, what has occurred wholesale across the UK has been the professionalization of teaching. Tutors in many UK universities are expected to hold a teaching qualification – even if many still do not have one – and tutors new to the university system are required to attend a mandatory programme in learning and teaching, usually provided by the university's in-house educational development unit. The consequences of this have not only been the elevation of the status of teaching and such development units, but also forms of innovative learning that are seen to promote particular capabilities in students, such as e-learning, autonomous learning and problem-based learning.

• *Facilitate observation.* One strategy for change is to provide tutors with an opportunity for direct observation of problem-based learning so that they are able to see how an innovative approach works. Direct observation seems to provide tutors with a new awareness that not all academic cultures are alike and that they do not all operate within the same instructional paradigm. Understanding differences in cultural context can help tutors to navigate within their own and make positive changes toward improvement.

- *Provide released time.* One of the major obstacles to change is time. Systematic course design is scholarly and intense work. This issue may be particularly important to tutors new to the approach, who may wonder whether the investment of their valuable time would benefit them as much in the promotion and tenure stakes as would undertaking traditional research instead. Investing in a more intensive approach to teaching is risky. Such scholarly work includes being content-current in one's field, understanding how the basic principles and concepts of one's field can be most effectively learned by students, determining valid and reliable means of assessing student learning and skilfully delivering the designed course. If change efforts are to be successful, tutor time must be understood and valued and released time can be a powerful motivator.

- *Offer rewards and incentives.* Rewards and incentives can provide opportunities, and encourage tutors to become involved in educational reform. Often, reward systems directly value tutors' research efforts rather than their strong commitment to teaching. This emphasis will need to change, as rewards given for outstanding teaching can create an environment of positive perception of this commitment. Finally, recognizing teaching in rewards systems makes a statement about the values of an institution; it says that teaching is valued here.

- *Encourage relationships with stakeholders.* One way to effect change is to bring in external stakeholders to encourage it. The larger community, such as business, industry, health service confederations and government, may have already called for change and it is important to respond to such calls if they are appropriate. In addition, connections with stakeholders may validate change even more, as its results are seen operating outside the university.

- *Support innovative assessment.* With ever-increasing calls for accountability and quality, assessment has great power to affect change. A regular programme of departmental outcomes assessment, including assessment of student learning and periodic review of the curriculum, can create opportunities for improvement.

- *Change traditional teaching evaluation approaches.* Traditional student evaluations of teaching tend to favour traditional teaching methods. They tend to ask questions like, 'Did the tutor present information clearly?' 'Was the tutor's presentation organized?' 'Was the teacher an effective lecturer?' Clearly these kinds of prompts favour traditional values and methods of teaching. Other forms of student evaluation, including more qualitative approaches to gather information, can provide additional light as to whether innovative approaches to teaching and learning such as problem-based learning are accomplishing their goals. In addition, while teaching evaluations provide one source of information, they are just that: one source. Evaluation of teaching should move beyond student evaluation and include other forms as well, to allow for multiple data points. Evaluation should be done for formative (for improvement) as well as summative purposes (for accountability).

Conclusion

As we have shown in this chapter, there are many levels of culture to consider when implementing change, which include national, disciplinary, institutional and individual cultures. Implementing change within these frameworks, bound together by shared assumptions, values and patterns of behaviour, can be quite challenging. The idea of effecting a dramatic or radical change from a traditional teaching paradigm to an active learning paradigm such as problem-based learning should be approached with knowledge and awareness of the nature of change being attempted and the academic culture into which it is being introduced. Attempts at change will be more successful if appropriate structures are in place to guide change.

In Part 1 of this book, we considered some conceptual frames of problem-based learning. In so doing, we raised myriad issues and questions. The question arises, for example, as to where problem-based learning fits within the different learning theories and learning traditions. Perhaps the question is moot. There really is no one correct learning theory and many of these theories share common characteristics and overlap with others, so why should we limit ourselves to one? Problem-based learning is a complex approach to learning and because of this perhaps combinations and balance serve us better. For us, there are no narrowly defined characteristics of problem-based learning. Instead there are people working in contexts using problem-based approaches. Problem-based learning is an approach to learning that is affected by the structural and pedagogical environment into which it is placed, in terms of the discipline or subject, the faculty and the organization concerned. It is to these differences that we turn in Part 2.

Part II

Recurring themes

6

What is a problem?

Introduction

The issue of what might count as a problem and the complexity of problem design is something that is a challenge to many tutors implementing problem-based learning. Some people design the problems themselves; others use templates or download problems that can be adapted. There are problem-based learning programmes available to buy, complete with all the problems. However, in every approach, there are still questions to be answered and additions to be made. In this chapter we examine what might count as a problem and explore some related literature. We suggest that it is important to consider how problems are used within a course or programme, and that problems should be designed not only to encourage students in the use of different types of knowledge and capabilities but also to motivate and keep motivating them.

What is a problem?

To date, much of the discussion in the field of problem-based learning about the nature of problems has centred on literature in cognitive psychology. For example, there have been discussions about the role of problem solving in problem-based learning and whether problem solving is a generalizable skill or not. While the cognitive science literature offers useful guidance, which we discuss below, the issue about what might count as a problem in problem-based learning relates rather less to the cognitive end of problem-solving literature and rather more to the issues about what it is that we want students to learn.

There is a further problem too in understanding what it is we are asking students to do. Are we asking them to solve a closed problem by using linear problem-solving techniques? Or are we asking them to do something very different, such as using their experiential and propositional knowledge to manage a problem situation? These are two very different activities and if students do not understand what is expected of them then the kind of scenario below can result:

> *It is Monday morning, 8.45, and the door of the design studio bursts open. Tim and Bill rush over to Jack to tell him that they have cracked the problem scenario. The group have been working on the problem all weekend but struggled, until now, to figure it out. The two who have found a way of managing the problem scenario share their views with the others. The group is oblivious to the tutor until he comes over to tell them that they have got the wrong answer. They are defeated, deflated and distraught that they have worked so hard for no result. Tim remains unconvinced that they are wrong and while the tutor gives the class a mini lecture he sits and works it all out again. At the end of the session, the group argue with the tutor who discovers, through this group, that there are in fact several ways to solve this particular problem.*
>
> (Savin-Baden 2000: 1)

What we see here is the assumption, by the students, that the problem they were expected to engage with was open-ended and that there were a variety of ways of solving it. The tutor on the other hand had designed the problem as one that required particular knowledge to solve, and he expected students to use a linear problem-solving approach to reach the same answer as him, and in the same way. The difficulty occurred when students challenged his narrow approach to problem-based learning. In this case the tutor was prepared to discuss the students' solution with them, but other tutors might have just assumed that the students were wrong. Thus the difficulty about what counts as a problem not only relates to problem design but also about how we expect students to engage with it.

Transferring knowledge and skills?

Many of the arguments for adopting problem-based learning in order to educate students for the professions stem from the idea that it will help students to transfer knowledge from university to practice. This assumption is problematic. Studies in both psychology and medical education have found that transfer from one context to another is less frequent and more difficult than is generally believed. Furthermore, Eva *et al.* (1998) argue that the content of the problem and the problem-solving abilities required of the students are two different concerns:

> If there were only one way to solve a problem, it might indeed be possible to identify the relevant content, devise a test to measure it, then correlate it with the appropriate measure of problem-solving. Unfortunately for this purpose, there are many ways to solve a problem, ranging from a detailed analysis of the aspects of the content of the problem to a simple recognition that the problem has been encountered before.
>
> (Eva *et al.* 1998: S1)

They suggest that it is important to recognize that there are three dimensions to a problem

1   the context: the physical context of the problem and the implied task;
2   the content: the semantic domain such as the disciplinary areas of knowledge and the surface elements such as the clients' details;
3   the schema or deep structure: the underlying principle of the problem.

However, regardless of content or principles of problem solving, it is the context in which the initial problem is presented that tends to affect the degree to which transfer of knowledge takes place. For example, a student's ability to transfer knowledge gained in one problem situation to another will be affected by whether the student expects the principles used in solving the two problems to be related. Schoenfeld (1985) showed that students trained on a geometry problem did not transfer their knowledge to solving construction problems because they believed that such problems should be solved using trial and error. However, Eva *et al.* suggest that transfer of knowledge between problems of the same domain (such as chest pain) is much more likely when the context has changed. This means that we should give students the opportunity to practise solving similar problems in the classroom; in this case an example would be different clients with various types of chest pain.

In order to improve transfer Eva *et al.* suggest that it is important to:

• teach problem recognition so that students can see the similarities between problems of different domains;
• provide immediate feedback and guidance;
• emphasize the importance of problem solving as a valuable learning tool;
• provide numerous examples so that students are able to understand abstract principles.

Problem design

One of the difficulties of problem design that occurs in many curricula is that little attention is paid to the different types of problems available, how they might be used and the level of the curriculum where they are used. For example, in some medical programmes problems change in terms of complexity and capability as the students progress through the first two years of the programme, yet the level of criticality the students are expected to develop towards learning and knowledge often changes very little. The assumption in many programmes is that students will be able to recognize and describe knowledge and issues before, in the third year, they are able to defend and evaluate. Much of this stems from the over-use of, and over-emphasis on, the cognitive domain of Bloom's taxonomy in undergraduate programmes. Bloom (1956) identified six levels within the cognitive domain, from the simple recall or recognition of facts, at the lowest level, through increasingly more complex and abstract mental levels, to the highest order that is classified as evaluation. Verb examples that represent intellectual activity on each level, and that could be used in the wording of a problem scenario are listed below.

1   **Knowledge:** arrange, define, duplicate, label, list, memorize, name, order, recall, recognize, relate, repeat, reproduce, state.
2   **Comprehension:** classify, describe, discuss, explain, express, identify, indicate, locate, recognize, report, restate, review, select, translate.
3   **Application:** apply, choose, demonstrate, dramatize, employ, illustrate, interpret, operate, practice, schedule, sketch, solve, use, write.
4   **Analyse:** analyse, appraise, calculate, categorize, compare, contrast, criticize, differentiate, discriminate, distinguish, examine, experiment, question, test.
5   **Synthesis:** arrange, assemble, collect, compose, construct, create, design, develop, formulate, manage, organize, plan, prepare, propose, set up, write.
6   **Evaluation:** appraise, argue, assess, attach, choose, compare, defend, estimate, evaluate, judge, predict, rate, score, select, support, value.

Bloom's cognitive levels are useful when beginning to develop problems for students but the difficulty is that it is easy to become completely centred on this approach and thus the problem-based learning becomes epistemologically focused. Problem-based learning problems should engage the student as a whole being but it is important to note that in integrated problem-based courses and programmes students are actually engaged in critical thinking almost as soon as they engage with problem-based learning. Barnett (1994) has suggested that approaches such as problem-based learning help students to develop independence in inquiry and to take up a stance towards knowledge. If students understand that they are to use critical thinking from Year 1 onwards, then they will see that engaging with the problem will not merely involve the application of a narrowly defined problem-solving skill to achieve a correct answer but instead will be a means of developing understanding of the subject. Barnett has argued for three levels of criticality, as follows:

Critical thinking

These are cognitive acts undertaken by the individual. Students engaged in critical thinking may do so in the company of other students and their critical thinking may be enhanced through that interchange; but the emphasis in the term critical thinking is on the character of the individual's cognitive acts.

Critical thought

This has a wider focus than just the individual's thought processes. Critical thought is collaborative and takes place within the discipline of study. For example, individuals might be doing some hard critical thinking but critical thought develops and takes off through sustained interchange around collective perspectives. Critical thought necessarily contains a social component and thus can only be developed collaboratively.

Critique

Critique is a form of criticism about the discipline itself, seeking to set it in a wider context rather than merely having internal debates within the discipline. In critique, different views of an issue or situation may be proffered as alternative perspectives are taken on board. This is a real cognitive and personal challenge, and it may open up the way to a transformation of the individual student.

By using Barnett's levels of critical thought we can design problems for the first year that help develop critical thinking, in the second year critical thought and thence in the third year, critique, as in Table 6.1. We would argue these could be transposed into the curriculum, enabling students to develop their critical capabilities as well as their skills and knowledge.

In his later writing Barnett has argued for the development, through higher education, of a critical being (Barnett 1997, 2000). The proposed model is based on an understanding of modern curricula being an educational project that forms the student as a critical being with three interlinking identities founded in the domains of knowledge, action and self (as discussed in Chapter 4). Thus in order to inspire the development of criticality within our students we need to begin by designing problems in ways that engage students with different levels of criticality. That is not to say that critique cannot take place earlier in the programme but it does mean that

Table 6.1 Progressive criticality

	Level of criticality	Features	Type of problem
Year 1	Critical thinking	Development of autonomy Use reasoning, analysis and synthesis	Task focused, but enables students to both develop personal autonomy and also work collaboratively
Year 2	Critical thought	Collective learning and action Critical dialogue	Moral problems that demand learning with and through the team: dialogic learning
Year 3	Critique	Criticism of the discipline Taking a stance towards knowledge	Problems of complexity that encourage students to critique the knowledge of the discipline and contest the discipline itself

the problems should centre on the development of criticality in the students rather than on a staged model such as that offered by Bloom.

Types of knowledge or types of problem?

At a recent workshop tutors attempted to define the difference between an undergraduate final-year problem and a master's level problem. The difficulties they experienced stemmed not only from their understanding of what counted as a complex problem, but also the way in which the learning experiences of the students would impact upon their ability to engage with the problem. For example, if the final-year students had been learning through problem-based learning since the first year of their programme they would be experienced 'problem-managers'. In contrast, many of those commencing a master's programme might have little or no experience of problem-based learning.

Early work by Schmidt and Bouhuijs (1980) defined problems in a typology that distinguished between the types of material presented to students. These were:

1   problems;
2   strategy tasks;
3   action tasks;
4   discussion tasks;
5   study tasks.

Table 6.2 links these to types of problems that may be used in problem-based learning.

To date there has been little research on the impact of the different types of problems on students' experiences of problem-based learning, nor has there been much exploration of the use of the different types of problem at different levels of the course. However, the taxonomy of problems developed by Schmidt and Moust (2000a) is a useful guide. Schmidt and Moust base their taxonomy on the assumptions that

Table 6.2 Problem typology

Stimulus material	
Problems	Problems of explanation: 'What is going on here?'
Strategy tasks	'What if' task. 'What would you do?'
Action tasks	Doing an activity, for example, interviewing business leaders
Discussion tasks	Tasks that focus on students' opinions
Study tasks	Tasks that can be done by an individual and do not require group discussion

Based on Schmidt and Bouhuijs (1980)

- students acquire different categories of knowledge during their course of study;
- different problem types will guide students towards these different categories.

As Schmidt and Moust note, limited attention has been given to the design of problems for problem-based learning. However, they do suggest that there are many descriptions of attributes of problems in the social psychology literature, such as complexity, concreteness and familiarity. What is both interesting and useful about this taxonomy is the focus of using problems to acquire different kinds of knowledge rather than solving problems or covering subject matter.

The work undertaken by Schmidt and Moust (2000a) is important not only for the way they provide and explicate different problem types, but also for their exploration of the way in which the questions asked of students guide the types of knowledge in which they engage. For example, the question, 'What is the matter with this man?' results in students seeking explanatory knowledge; knowledge that offers some reason for the symptoms the man is experiencing. Whereas if the students were asked, 'What would you do if you were this man's physiotherapist?' then the emphasis becomes one of action rather than explanation. Thus the assumption is that the student always understands the explanatory knowledge and can take action, thereby using procedural knowledge. Such a distinction is important because it helps students to begin to understand how they recognize and use different types of knowledge.

It is important for students to realize that there are different forms of knowledge, and that an understanding of different forms can help them both when learning at university and in life in general. Different theorists have argued for different types of knowledge and some of these differ while others overlap with one another. What we would suggest here is that in problem-based learning a starting point would be to make students understand the differences between objective knowledge, personal knowledge and procedural knowledge. For example, if students understand that objective knowledge is what is produced and recorded by researchers, but that such knowledge also needs to be critiqued and questioned, this will help them to understand that not all research is necessarily good research. If students understand that personal knowledge, representing people's attitudes and values, is more difficult to critique than objective knowledge, this will help them to see both the importance and challenges of their own moral perspectives on issues. Furthermore, students also need to understand that descriptive knowledge can pose further challenges, such as the difficulty that although descriptive knowledge comprises facts it also includes things we may comprehend but find difficult to explain. For example, taking a daily aspirin is currently seen to reduce the possibility of a heart attack but why this is the case is currently unclear from research and experience. However, students also need to engage with fact-finding problems, such as, 'What is the judicial system in South Africa?' since it will help them to find out about courts, laws and the South African legal system. Recognition of different kinds of knowledge can help students to realize that different problems may require the application of those different types of knowledge, as demonstrated in Table 6.3.

Schmidt and Moust suggest that such a taxonomy is useful in the first two years of a programme but that more complex problems in the third year will involve combining the types of problems shown in the Table 6.3. However, they also note that the purpose of the problem is contained more often in the instructions given to the students rather than in the text of the problems.

The challenges of problem design

In Chapter 4 we discussed different curricula models and here we suggest that the type of model adopted can have an impact on the types of problems that can be utilized within a given curriculum. However, before we discuss this further, there are two other difficulties that need consideration. First, it is our experience that many tutors set out to design problems that are based only on the content that they feel their students need to cover. In practice what occurs is that a decision is made to turn the whole programme into a problem-based one. Then tutors meet together a number of times to decide just how much knowledge can be crammed into such a programme and what each module or course is going to cover. Next, tutors take away the list of knowledge to be covered and design problems to fit around this list. At quite a basic level this can work quite well as it is easy to see where students are covering each component of knowledge and it seems to be a simple way of covering the knowledge base that students are expected to acquire. The difficulty with this approach is that the focus is still very much on students learning pre-prescribed chunks of knowledge, it is still highly tutor-directed and it gives students little choice about what it is they learn. The starting point for designing problems should not be the knowledge base or the type and level of skills but rather the capabilities that students need to develop that will equip them for working in a shifting and complex world.

Some time ago a story was told at a conference. The speaker suggested that by the time we left at the end of his hour-long session 10 per cent of what we had learned would no longer be up to date, and that in a year's time at the end of an hour's lecture 40 per cent of what we had learned would not be up to date. Thus in five years' time students would go into a lecture theatre and what was up to date during the lecture would be out of date by the time they came out of it! This may be just anecdotal but there is a point. What students need to develop are capabilities for knowledge retrieval and management, and skill development, rather than attending sessions that involve them in just covering vast amounts of propositional knowledge. Developing a curriculum that enables this to happen may be challenging and so may developing problems for such a curriculum, but this is what we need to do to equip our students.

Table 6.3 Types of knowledge and types of problems

Types of knowledge	Explanatory knowledge	Descriptive knowledge	Procedural knowledge	Personal knowledge
Types of problems	Explanation problem	Fact-finding problem	Strategy problem	Moral dilemma problem
Examples	People in the 15th century used to believe it was possible to fall off the edge of the earth.	Following recent political changes relating to land use in Zimbabwe, many internal borders have changed.	A 43-year-old woman cannot lift her right arm more than 45 degrees and she complains of pins and needles in her hand.	A mother breaks into a chemist's shop at night to obtain life-saving drugs for her baby. She contacts her local physician the next day to explain what she has done.
Example of question	Explain why.	What would a legal map look like?	If you were this client's physiotherapist what would you do?	What should the doctor do?

(Adapted from Schmidt and Moust 2000: 68)

The second difficulty in problem design is that few tutors consider the type or the level of the problems that they are designing. Although it is quite difficult to offer a generic typology of problems that fit all disciplines, subjects and progressions, there is considerable mileage in such a typology because it does at least help us to focus on the simplicity and complexity of the problems we are asking students to consider. It also challenges us to ask ourselves why we are putting particular types of problems in given areas of the programme. There is often a sense that the more complicated a problem and the more difficult the level of knowledge the later in the programme it should appear, so that students only undertake complicated problems in the final year of their programme. Yet complicated problems are not just for final-year students and what appears complicated to one tutor may be easy to another. For some tutors this might mean moral dilemmas, for another it might be dealing with a client with multiple injuries, and for others it might mean engaging with a different cultural context.

Problems that motivate students to learn

When designing problems it is essential to consider the balance between discipline knowledge and process skills such as problem solving and teamwork. When introducing problem-based learning to students for the first time it is often helpful to start students off with a problem scenario that is fun, humorous and non-technical, in which they do not feel too threatened. For example:

> *You are a group of first-year students who have been given a project via University Enterprises. You have been asked to work with a firm who hold the patent for pedal bins and swing-top bins. The management team of this firm, having seen the high sales figures for the Dyson vacuum cleaner and new Dyson washing machine, has recently decided that these bins are not aesthetically pleasing nor ergonomically sound. This means that they expect such bins will not exist in the long term and they require you to design a new refuse accommodator. You have been given 20 minutes to come up with a strategy.*
>
> *The only other information you have been given is that this new product must sell and that it is expected that pedal bins and swing-top bins will be replaced in households worldwide within six months.*

This will enable students to focus on something other than just solving the problem – such as the development of group skills or a consideration of what learning means in this kind of context. Furthermore, we have also found that there are ways of writing and presenting problems so that students remain interested and do not become tired and bored with problem-based learning. These include:

- Start with a problem about which students will have some knowledge, this develops their confidence and enthusiasm.

- Use problems that will gain their interest, such as those relevant to practice. For example, we found that asking student midwives to learn about women's health was not something that motivated them, they wanted to know about health in pregnancy. The answer was to give them a problem relating to a healthy expectant mother so that they would learn about women's health, but in the context of something that was motivating to them.
- The problem should have a puzzle, mystery or some drama so that it is unclear at the start what is going on.
- Ensure that the problems are varied by using video clips, actors, answer-machine messages and different types of media presentation, and not just paper cases. Students belong to the soundbite generation and thus the presentation of material needs to reflect this.
- Wherever possible use authentic problems, situations from real life. Students quickly pick out situations that are not authentic and consequently they feel that they are being manipulated into learning rather than stimulated to explore their own agendas.

However, it is also important to ensure that when you are designing problems you develop a tutor guide to help facilitators, and that you review the problems with other tutors so that they can criticize the problems. Time spent checking problems at the outset saves much time later. When tutors are new to problem design three common mistakes are made. The first is not providing some sort of statement or question at the end of the problem. Students need this so that they have some sense of what is expected of them and which types of knowledge are required to deal with the problem. The second is making a problem too narrow so that students try to solve it in a simplistic and formulaic way. The third is producing over-complex problems. An example of an over-complex problem would be: an elderly man who is blind, has had both legs amputated, lives in a top-floor apartment with no lift and has been admitted to the local hospital's accident and emergency unit hearing voices.

Conclusion

Problem design is a complex and multifaceted issue about which there are relatively few straightforward answers. Due to the nature of knowledge within different disciplines and the fact that disciplines use knowledge differently, it is not possible to provide an exhaustive taxonomy of how to design problems for particular curricula. However, we do suggest that some consideration should be given to the types of problems used at different levels of the course and the types of questions that students are asked to engage with in the context of solving or managing a problem. Discussing types of knowledge, types of questions and the place of criticality in problems can help tutors to design problems that help students to explore their own views about what counts as knowledge and to understand what it is they need to learn both individually and collectively within the problem-based learning team.

7

Learning in teams

Introduction

One of the most frequently asked questions about problem-based learning is whether or not it must be done in teams. Many people have asked us about the relative importance of teams and why students in problem-based learning should be expected to work in teams. While some have recently begun to suggest that problem-based learning may be done with individuals, we support the team approach. We argue that in life, we invariably have to work in teams, yet there is little in our school and university systems that equip us for life in teams. Investment in team learning would seem to us to be a vital component of higher education, one that we should embrace, and problem-based learning can help us to do just that. This approach offers some distinct advantages over individual learning as well as some unique challenges, and this chapter outlines some of the advantages and characteristics of team learning and answers some practical questions and considerations about how to create successful teams.

Differences between learning teams and other types of teams

Students will have participated in a variety of teams prior to experiencing working in their first learning team, such as sports teams, religious groups, social clubs and music bands. However, few of these are formed for the primary purpose of learning. It is often felt that unless we make learning goals clear, maintain the essential components of learning teams, and provide students with structure and practice, they might gain little from the experience. However, much can also be gained through dialogue. For example, Jacobsen (1997) argued that discussion about problems and issues beyond the problem-based learning team were vital to enable learning to take place. Jacobsen termed these discussions frame factors, issues that students raised that do not directly relate to the problem scenario but are important to students. Examples of frame factors include transport between campuses, the arrival of student uniforms, the previous night's television, and students' personal problems.

Understanding learning in teams

Proponents of team learning use a variety of terms including collaborative learning, cooperative learning, action learning and team learning. Here we draw from a variety of sources to reach an understanding of what team learning can mean within the context of a problem-based learning environment. Thus to support our understanding of this concept we draw from the broader body of literature which takes as its focus learning in teams in academe. There are several models of team learning. The post-industrialist model describes the shift from hierarchically structured decision-making to the use of teamwork and consensus for problem solving. This model assumes that 'two heads or more are better than one' and thus will arrive at a better solution than any single individual can supply. The social constructivist model is based in theories of social constructivism; in which learners construct knowledge through discourse with other members of the community, including the tutor. Learning is produced by the team, and not reproduced from disciplinary authority. The popular democratic model is predicated on difference and thus takes account of the multicultural student environment. In this model, as Hamilton notes, 'the challenge is for instructors not to obliterate essential differences in the search for commonalties but rather to envision these essential differences of age, race, colour, economic status, background, motivation or prior knowledge as catalysts for the making of meaning within the specific concepts of the particular course' (Hamilton 1994: 95). These models have different epistemological underpinnings but share the common theme that working in teams is essential to the learning process. Much of what occurs in problem-based learning, however, tends to resemble the following types of teams:

1   the tutor-guided learning team;
2   the collaborative learning team;
3   the reflexive team;
4   the cooperative team;
5   the action learning team.

The tutor-guided learning team

The facilitator in this type of team sees his or her role as guiding the students through each component of the problem. Thus students see problem scenarios as being set within, or bounded by, a discrete subject or disciplinary area. In some situations, the tutor actually provides hints and tips on problem-solving techniques; the argument for such an approach is that students have limited skills to help them solve the problems they will encounter. The result is that students often see solutions as being linked to specific curricular content. This kind of approach follows a model proposed by Woods *et al.* (1975):

Definition of the problem

- The system. Students identify the system under study by analysing and interpreting the information available in a problem statement.
- Known(s) and concepts. Students list what they know about the problem.
- Unknown(s). Students list what they need to know about the problem.
- Units and symbols. Students select, interpret and use units and symbols needed to solve the problems.
- Constraints. Students look for limiting factors, or constraints in the problem.
- Criteria for success. Students determine what an appropriate type of response could look like.

Contemplation and research

- Simmering. Students ponder the problem.
- Identification of specific pieces of knowledge. Students identify the required background information necessary to solve the problem.
- Collection of information. Students collect pertinent information they need to solve the problem.

Planning a solution

- Possible strategies. Students review the broader structure of the problem and some potential strategies for a solution.
- Best strategy. Students choose the best strategy for problem solving.

Carry out the plan

- Students carry out their plan, being patient and persistent.

Reflection and evaluation

- Students review their solutions.

- Students ask themselves whether the answer makes sense, whether the solution meets the criteria, and whether their solution is viable.
- Students reflect on their learning considering whether they could have done better.

Interestingly, the premise here is that the tutor's role in teaching these skills is essential, so issues of who is in control of the learning are not negotiated. Tutors are in control; they have power over the content and the process.

The collaborative learning team

This is probably the most common form of learning seen in problem-based tutorials. Although it could be viewed as largely based on models of collaborative inquiry, an element of tutor control still exists. For example, the focus is on the development of specific levels of skills and thus small-team social skills are essential for successful collaboration in the problem-based learning environment. In addition to being able to communicate clearly with, accept and support all other team members individually as well as resolve conflicts, students must be able to elicit each other's viewpoints and perspectives, question each other's assumptions and evidence, make decisions, manage the 'business' of the team and often make presentations to the larger year group. Bosworth (1994: 27) developed the following taxonomy of collaborative skills, and also suggests (pp. 30–1) strategies to teach them:

- *Identification:* Observe students during the first week of the module and note areas of strength and weakness. Alternatively, engage the students themselves in evaluation by videotaping 5–10 minutes of the team working together on a task. Facilitate the team reviewing the tape together so that members can identify essential skills.
- *Demonstration of skills:* Pose examples of the skill as it might be used in a team setting, such as a role-play demonstrating the skill.
- *Modelling:* Model the skill and explain what you are doing and why. Break the whole task down and demonstrate the steps in keeping a team on task: define the task, set and agree the agenda, set a timeframe, monitor the time and progress, and remind each other of what needs to be done.
- *Performance feedback:* Tutors or students can give feedback. At the end of a session, have the team evaluate the effectiveness of a skill.
- *Reflection:* Give students the opportunity to talk about their experiences and discuss how they can improve their skills. Develop a self-evaluation questionnaire to guide students' reflections.

Tutors often believe that students' lack of collaborative skills will necessarily be problematic, especially when they start problem-based learning. However, who defines which collaborative skills are valuable is largely based on a view of students' conformity to tutor perspectives, and these can vary from team to team. For many students, being adequately prepared to complete their assigned tasks successfully is what is at the heart of this approach, and thus it is deemed the tutor's responsibility to take the time to teach students to be successful team members.

The reflexive team

This kind of learning team is largely based in cooperative models of problem-based learning and Freireian forms of pedagogy (Freire 1972, 1974). For example, in this type of team, working together is often talked about in terms of a journey but it is seen as less stable, less convergent and less collaborative than the existing literature relating to groups and group theory would imply. Reflexivity here is seen as an organizing principle, and thus it involves explicit shared reflection about the team process and findings of the learning needs of the team, rather than the masking of the kinds of paradoxes and conflicts that emerge at almost every stage in most learning teams. Students in such teams are expected to feel able to point to unease connected both with their role within the team, the relationship between their individual concerns (that may stand in direct conflict with the collective ethos of the team), and the nature of support within the team. In these types of teams, therefore, each member is valued, the optimum setting is created for ideas to grow, and individuals are empowered through affirmation. Thus the team serves as an interactive function for the individual. Through the team, the individual is enabled to learn both through the experience of others and the appreciation of other people's life-worlds; and by reflecting upon these, to relate them to their own. Thus individual students, by making themselves and their learning the focus of reflection and analysis within the team, are able to value alternative ways of knowing. Dialogue here is central to progress in people's lives, and it is through dialogue that values are deconstructed and reconstructed, and experiences relived and explored, in order to make sense of roles and relationships.

The cooperative team

In an extensive meta-analysis that included hundreds of studies, Johnson *et al.* (1991) concluded that collaborative learning arrangements were superior to competitive, individualistic structures on a variety of outcomes such as higher academic achievement, higher-level reasoning, more frequent generation of new ideas and solutions, and greater transfer of learning from one situation to another. The difference between cooperative learning and collaborative learning is that cooperative learning involves small group work to maximize student learning. This approach tends to maintain traditional lines of knowledge and authority whereas collaborative learning is based on notions of social constructivism. As Matthews puts it 'it (collaborative learning) is a pedagogy that has at its centre the assumption that people make meaning together and that the process enriches and enlarges them' (Matthews 1995: 101).

Cooperative learning is appropriate whenever the goals of learning are highly important, mastery and retention are important, the task is complex or conceptual, problem solving, divergent thinking or creativity is desired, quality of performance is expected and higher-level reasoning strategies and critical thinking are needed (Johnson *et al.* 1991: 40). These are skills particularly desired in the problem-based learning environment. In addition to the academic-cognitive abilities, social and emotional abilities also improve when students work in teams (Millis and Cottell 1998). Students are more likely to be successful if they make formal connections with other students in the context of academic work that they then carry into informal activities. In addition, compared with competitive learning environments, a more cooperative learning setting creates more positive relationships among a diverse team of students, students like each other and the tutor better, and students demonstrate more concern and social support for their peers (Slavin 1990; Johnson *et al.* 1998). Along with creating better academic, cognitive, social and emotional abilities for all students, a cooperative learning environment creates opportunities for those typically marginalized in traditional education. In particular, learning in teams can provide opportunities for women and minorities who are often not as likely to speak out in a competitive educational environment. Women and minority students report more favourable attitudes toward learning in teams than their white male counterparts, and research shows that team learning is more likely to improve learning in these categories of students (Treisman 1985; Cabrera 1998; Millar 1999).

The action learning team

Action learning is based on the idea, developed by Revans in the 1960s (Revans 1983), that through the process of reflection and action it is possible to solve problems. An action learning set is formed by a group of people coming together over a stated period of time with the aim of 'getting things done' (McGill and Beaty 2001: 1). In practice this means that when the set is formed each member brings a real-life problem to it that they want help in solving. Action learning is a form of learning based on the interrelationship of learning and action, and thus the learning occurs through a continuous process of reflecting and acting by the individual on their problem with the help of the learning set. The learning set is designed to be more than a straightforward support group, because the role of all other set members is to help individual members in dealing with their particular problem. However, a set is not a formal meeting with an agenda, nor is it a counselling group, nor a critical incident analysis to be undertaken over lunch. Instead it is a formalized process whereby the set meets on a regular basis to undertake action that will deal with or resolve problems, and thus the focus of the set is on the learning from the actions taken by the individual. Set lifespans tend to vary between six months and three years. The difference between problem-based learning and action learning is that the essence of an action learning set is its focus on the individual and their future action (McGill and Beaty 2001: 14–15). In problem-based learning, the team would normally function by seeking to achieve the tasks collaboratively. Using action learning sets as a learning approach for problem-based learning centres the power more on students than the tutor. It will result in a more individualized group of team members, freer flowing interaction and be centred more upon personal learning and reflection in order to achieve effective action than would be seen in a collaborative group process.

The advantages of students working in learning teams

Team learning provides students with the opportunity to work together. They know that they will have to work with others in the community and in their job, and learning the essential skills to function successfully in these situations while in a safe environment is a real advantage. As one tutor we know eloquently puts it to his students: 'There is no job in the world where your boss will lecture to you for 50 minutes as you frantically take notes to later give you a test in which you regurgitate the information. Working in problem-based teams is something you will have to do in the real world and you may as well learn to do it now.' Team learning also provides opportunities for students to network, exchange ideas and information, and value diverse opinions. The numerous studies that have been conducted on learning in teams indicate that there are a number of outcomes that team learning improves. Perhaps first among the outcomes authors most often note is improved cognitive and academic outcomes (Millis and Cottell 1998). Students perhaps learn best through teaching other students (McKeachie 1994), and working in teams gives learners the opportunity to articulate their knowledge, thus owning it in a different way. Learners must go even beyond articulation and put knowledge in such a way that they can then teach it to others. Astin (1993) notes that student learning in teams is superior to learning in other types of environments, perhaps because students are more actively engaged in the learning process.

Components of successful learning teams

Advocates of collaborative, cooperative or team learning argue that there are several essential components for effective learning teams (Johnson *et al.* 1998):

- *Positive interdependence,* meaning that team members need each other to succeed. All members of the team must be involved and committed to team success, although it could be argued that a larger team could still be successful even if there were a passenger or two in the team.
- *Promotive interactions,* implying that interaction between and among team members should be designed to promote the members and the team. Team members help each other, provide feedback for ongoing improvement and encourage an atmosphere of openness to diversity and new ideas.
- *Individual accountability,* indicating that even though functioning and normally being assessed on team processing and performance, individual students must be held accountable for their work and on their individual contributions to the team.
- *Teamwork and social skills,* achieving team functioning as effectively as possible, including decision-making, trust-building, communication and conflict management.
- *Team processing,* meaning undertaking reflection as a team at the conclusion of a problem in order to identify their strengths and weaknesses and ensuring improvement next time.

Ideal team size

Advocates of the team approach have diverse opinions about optimal team size, and these often depend on the nature of the task. Some prefer to keep teams small to maximize student involvement and participation and recommend teams of two to three. However, smaller teams can have personality conflicts and may not achieve maximum diversity. Most recommend having enough team members who can combine their diversity of talents and experience to deal with the problem. In a problem-based learning environment, with the learning catalyst being a complex problem, this most often means a team of at least five. Teams of four may tend to form two pairs, and teams of three may form a pair and an outsider; five seems to be sufficient to allow for team cohesion (Bruffee 1999). Most people using problem-based learning would suggest that teams of eight are ideal; although this is not often easily achievable in most universities today.

Managing membership

The general consensus in the literature is to allow the tutor to determine team membership to achieve maximum heterogeneity for long-term teams (Johnson *et al.* 1991). However, this does raise issues about team ownership and the tutor's power within and over the team. It is important to remember that diversity can represent a variety of characteristics such as age, ethnicity, experience, academic abilities and capabilities. Permitting students to form their own teams can lead to teams based on friendship and again, may not allow for maximum diversity, which limits students' ability to learn from as many viewpoints as possible. It has been suggested that, during short breaks out of long-term teams, allowing students to work with peers whose company they enjoy can have benefits (Brookfield and Preskill 1999), while random selection can provide the appearance of fairness. Short breaks out can maximize student networking and experiences in working with a wide variety of students.

Roles and ground rules

Very few students come to higher education with well-developed team skills. To function in teams, they will need a range of skills and abilities that include interpersonal skills, active learning, team building and management, inquiry skills, conflict skills and presentation skills (Bosworth 1994). If students are new to problem-based learning, they may not have had opportunities to function within teams, nor will they be familiar with the kinds of activities and functions that one may perform in a team setting. These students in particular, and all students in general, benefit from induction programmes and team building exercises (see, for example, King 2001).

Anyone who has been part of a team knows just how hard it can be to get all the members dedicated and motivated. Achieving team motivation demands commitment, and what underpins this is that the whole team must believe in the value of both teamwork itself and the task being undertaken. Problem-based learning can be implemented for a whole host of reasons (see for example Savin-Baden 2000), and invariably opportunities for team building are the first things to be erased from a curriculum due to a perception that there is inadequate time for content delivery. This is often the first step towards breakdown in teams. Teams need to be built, they need secure foundations, and at the outset they need to be clear about their own aims and goals in relation to the overarching curriculum expectations. Simultaneously, individual members of the team need to be clear about their own roles: why they are there and what is expected of them. Building teams in the first instance will help members to develop a sense of commitment that will sustain them through demanding periods of growth and development. Yet in our fragmented and incoherent society, there are difficulties with notions of commitment and teamwork. The shifts towards self-directed learning, autonomous learning and students as 'consumers' tends to promote a notion of individualism that signals an end to dialogue and with it a devaluing of collaborative and dialogic approaches to learning. This is culturally reinforced by government, industry and health services among others, who concentrate on meeting targets, which often bring with them a focus on outputs rather than outcomes, and the task rather than the process. Yet both an elected government and collections of ward staff need to learn to work together as effective teams.

Teams are motivated when they can see a value, purpose and sense of reality in their task. Therefore, task and process in problem-based learning teams need to be inextricably linked to real-world situations that will secure students' inquisitiveness and offer them feedback on their overall effectiveness. Nevertheless, it is often the case in health sciences curricula that students are expected to learn about 'the normal person' before they are permitted to explore disease and illness. The paradox is that the motivation of most students on such courses is to learn about illness – that is what they feel that they are there for. Students can learn about what counts as normal in the process of exploring illness. To do this will engage students' motivations that in turn will enhance team commitment.

Teams are also motivated by feedback and reward yet few problem-based seminars are rewarded in real terms. Students need to see their assessment as part of their learning process as well as part of their development towards being effective health professionals who can work in teams. Additionally, in order to ensure team commitment, students need to work together through a team-building activity to develop ground rules to which they all feel able to be bound and committed. Such ground rules can form the basis of a 'contract' between team members. The following example of a team learning contract emerged from a collaborative team building exercise:

1 The team will be committed to its membership in ways that will encourage sharing of information and realistic self-appraisal of the team and of individuals within it.
2 The team will create a safe and supportive learning context that promotes trust and commitment within the team.
3 Team members will give and receive feedback towards one another which is supportive and constructively critical.
4 Confidentiality of issues shared and discussed within the problem-based learning team will be maintained within the bounds of the team itself.
5 There will be a commitment to punctuality as defined by the team.
6 The team will develop its own commitment to attendance and decide upon ways in which it will manage non-attendance by its members.
7 The team will utilize self-regulation mechanisms as a means of ensuring equity is maintained across the team in terms of status, workload and contribution to the team.
8 Respect for contributions made by other members both verbally and in writing will be maintained as far as possible.
9 Team members will produce agreed work (as decided by the team) on time.
10 The team should seek to clarify, and contribute to, the definition of the role of the facilitator in the team.
11 The team should take shared responsibility for the progress of the process and outcomes of the team.
12 Team members should be willing to share knowledge with and learn from other members of their team.

Conclusion

Much of undergraduate learning at university focuses on outcomes that are predictable, whereas learning through teams is a means of educating people to learn with complexity. Learning in teams can help students to see that learning and life take place in contexts, contexts that affect the kinds of solutions that are available and possible. Learning in teams is not about developing a particular tool kit or set of strategies, from which it is possible to choose and then slot in the right one at the right time. Instead it demands that we recognize that learning occurs in a context, a time and a space, and that it is influenced by what the individual brings to the learning situation. In addition to issues we have presented, continual evaluation and feedback is essential for student success in problem-based learning. Students will have to work in teams in their communities and in their professions. Thus, working in teams while in academe builds bridges between personal and professional worlds and between propositional and practical knowledge. However, it is vital that students understand their roles in teams and are equipped to work in problem-based learning teams and it is to this that we turn next.

Table 7.1 Taxonomy of collaborative skills

Skill category	Small team collaborative skills
Interpersonal skills	Be congenial and friendly
	Make clear statements
	Listen
	Communicate positively (no name calling/put downs)
	Maintain eye contact
Team building/ management	Organize work
	Keep team on task
	Run a meeting
	Participate in team self-analysis
	Show empathy
Inquiry skills	Clarify
	Critique
	Probe assumptions and evidence
	Probe implications and consequences
	Elicit viewpoints and perspectives
Conflict	Prevent
	Resolve
	Mediate
Presentation	Summarize, synthesize
	Speak in front of a team
	Create presentation materials
	Write reports

8

The role of students

Introduction

Problem-based learning is often a new experience for students and calls for a change in student perspectives and functioning in any given programme. In this chapter we address the range of roles and responsibilities that students face in problem-based learning. The chapter begins as we explore the shift in student perspectives from traditional teaching to problem-based learning. We next outline key roles that individual students may assume in problem-based learning, followed by the team roles that they can undertake. We finally examine the place of conflict and the impact of a student's interactional stance on teamwork.

Shifts in perspectives

A dramatic shift comes in moving from a traditional lecture theatre to a problem-based learning experience. Students have shifted from one primary role (listener and observer) to a multitude of overlapping and ever-changing roles. They have shifted from one primary responsibility (learn the content) to a host of new responsibilities. Traditional paths of success have been changed; students know how to win the old game, but the new game has new rules. Traditional lines of authority have been called into question; no longer is the lecturer the comforting and all-knowing sage. Traditional conventions of privacy have been altered; no longer can the student conceal under-preparation or gaps in knowledge. Traditional lines of responsibility have been altered; no longer is the student a free agent; rather, she is responsible to her teammates.

Questions abound such as, 'I got straight As previously; will problem-based learning change that? Will I look stupid in front of my classmates? Am I really learning anything? Why won't the tutor just teach me? Will my team members pull their weight, or will I have to do all of the work? Will I be able to pass my professional examinations after this course – will I learn the content I need? Why should I have to do all of this work?' It is indeed natural for students to experience some apprehension and even some resistance. It is important to let them own these feelings, but it is equally important to address the anxiety before it gets out of hand. Providing students with information about the intent of problem-based learning and how it has been successful in the past can help alleviate some concerns. If tutors build trust into the learning environment and allow students the opportunity both to get to know each other and work in some low-threat situations then this can also help assuage distress. Research shows (Albanese and Mitchell 1993) that students who have experience of problem-based learning prefer it to traditional courses and that this preference increases with more exposure to the approach.

One of the most fundamental shifts that occurs when moving towards learner-centred philosophies is in understanding how students learn. An approach that focuses on learning, Barr and Tagg (1995) assert, suggests that knowledge exists in each person's mind, is shaped by individual experience and is constructed and created. Learning is a nesting and interacting of frameworks, is student-centred and controlled and is collaborative. This view of learning, they assert, is directly tied to and dramatically alters the roles that both tutors and students will assume. Students actively construct knowledge, they compare new knowledge with previous information, they share the responsibility with each other and they work in teams with each other and with tutors. These changes are evident in problem-based learning, where students make several dramatic shifts as follows:

- from passive listener, observer and note taker to active problem solver, contributor and discussant;
- from a private persona taking few or no risks to a public person who takes many risks;
- from attendance dictated by personal choice to attendance dictated by community expectation;
- from competition with peers to collaborative work with them;
- from responsibilities and self-definition associated with learning independently to those associated with learning interdependently; and
- from seeing tutors and texts as the sole sources of authority and knowledge to seeing peers, oneself and the community as additional and more important sources of authority and knowledge (adapted from MacGregor 1990).

Individual roles and responsibilities

Students in the problem-based learning environment will assume a variety of roles and responsibilities while undertaking a series of problems that are vastly different from those few they have assumed in traditional education. A particular student may find the subject matter of the first problem with which he is presented to be either his favourite or least favourite, so he will tend to assume the role either of expert or apprentice, respectively. During another problem scenario he may find himself being a passionate advocate for another team member's solution, in the face of most other team members' preference for a different solution. There follows a list of individual roles that students at any given time may assume. They can of course undertake more than one role at the same time.

Practical, real-world problem-solver

As a problem serves as the context and stimulus for learning, a student in a problem-based course serves first as a practical problem-solver. The context is dictated by the problem, which may well form an identity for the student to assume when solving the problem (for example a physician facing a challenging patient situation, educational leader meeting a worried board, biologist grappling with the problem of global warming). In this stakeholder role, consistent with a role the student might find herself assuming in the future, she solves a problem that someone in the role might face. It is in this role that a student analyses the situation, identifies the overarching structure of the problem and develops viable solutions to the problem.

Expert or decision-maker

The student serves as an expert in some areas of solving the problem, and working with other students allows each student the opportunity to assume such a role. A student analyses the situation in order to make a variety of decisions and identifies the learning issues within a given situation. The student may also suggest team member assignments and appraise the credibility of the information shared in team sessions.

Self-directed learner

In problem-based learning, the student takes an active, independent approach to learning by determining which issues to pursue and directing their own inquiry. Self-directed learning is a process in which individuals take the initiative to diagnose their learning needs, formulate learning goals, identify resources for learning, select and implement learning strategies and evaluate learning outcomes (Knowles 1978). A self-directed learner controls both the objectives and the means of learning (Mocker and Spear 1982). Self-directed learners are independent, self-motivated individuals who set clear goals, plan ahead, seek challenges and push normal limits to achieve high standards.

Communicator, educator or humanist

A problem-based learning student takes prior or new knowledge and communicates it to the other students in the team. In communicating with others, team members acknowledge differences of opinion and other perspectives. As communicators students demonstrate active listening and appropriate verbal and non-verbal behaviour. They respect others' opinions and allow everyone the opportunity to express themselves. They acknowledge the value of other members' contributions. Students participate in discussion of differences in moral values and rather than sweeping difficult issues under the carpet they have opportunities to explore them head on. They learn to differentiate value of information from value of person. Students work to negotiate differences and misunderstandings among team members, attempting to find resolution. They learn to speak effectively and directly to the team and present their ideas clearly and concisely, communicating in a language that their peers understand.

Advocate

Students in problem-based learning teams become advocates, pleading a cause for a client, defending a stance or a cause, or encouraging team members to agree with a position or with new information. They are prepared to offer representation, help and advice to constituents of the problem and to fellow team members. This role may involve conflict resolution, support, mediation and facilitation. The advocate interprets rules and policies in an attempt to recommend a sound solution to a question, issue or problem.

Participator in a community of learners

In a problem-based learning course, students not only assume some of the responsibility for their own learning, but also share in the responsibility for the learning of their fellow team members. As a participator in a community of learners, a student works to develop meaningful ways to enhance, enrich and celebrate other team members. Students seek and share learning and then act on what they have learned. They become learning communities, designed to engage in continuous inquiry and problem-solving. As members of the community, they engage in supportive and shared leadership, collective creativity, shared values and vision, supportive conditions and shared personal practice (Hord 1997).

Scientist or scholar

In the process of dealing with the problem, students become producers of knowledge who are capable of making significant contributions to the field's knowledge base. Students develop strong background knowledge in order to solve the problem. They establish clear goals to guide their direction and use appropriate procedures for investigation and inquiry. They obtain significant results and are given opportunities to reflect on their findings.

Apprentice

A problem-based learning student serves in the role of apprentice. This role occurs almost by proxy, as a student observes and applies the thinking processes used by practitioners in a particular field or discipline. Students also become tutors themselves by transmitting what they have learned to other students in the team.

Explorer

In a problem-based learning course, students interact with the physical world and with other people as they discover concepts and apply skills. They are often daring risk-takers as they engage in a new problem and explore possible solutions. They engage in 'out-of-the-box' thinking. They have time to reflect upon their discoveries and compare them with existing knowledge.

Creative and critical thinker

As creative thinkers, students come to problems and solutions with original and inventive ideas and solutions. They are inquisitive throughout the process. As critical thinkers, students analyse information by clarifying and setting the purpose and then selecting a strategy to achieve the purpose. They also process information, which they do through applying knowledge, making connections and formulating questions. They also evaluate information, monitor and manage learning and revise purpose and strategy when appropriate.

Person or individual

Students do not lose track of themselves and they work to clarify their values, abilities, interests and goals to other students. They seek to become self-aware and thus more proficient in self-evaluation. Students thus identify their own strengths and weaknesses as well as the means for resolving or correcting any deficiencies. Students, therefore, will be able to respond to constructive criticism without a grudge and by making changes when appropriate.

Mature adult

Students own their obligations and responsibilities and regularly attend team sessions on time. It is expected that they will be well prepared having completed their work as previously agreed with their team, and that they accept responsibility for their decisions and the work produced by the teams.

Gatekeeper or resource manager

Students will share equally responsibilities that facilitate their learning. They can assist each other by recording the learning issues, assumptions and connections made by the team, as well as other public lists of data or graphic representations important to their learning. They can moderate team sessions, keeping track of the time used to ensure the various and necessary activities of teamwork occur. They can also generate, find and share important resources for solving the problem. They demonstrate respect for each other and for materials that they use to pursue learning. Students use only the resources and materials that are necessary for the learning issue, sharing them with their fellow students and returning them when work is completed.

Team roles

In addition to the individual roles just mentioned, there are other roles that must be taken on by members to ensure that their team functions effectively. Team roles most often used in problem-based learning include:

- *facilitator*, who moderates discussions, keeps the team on task and makes sure everyone works and has the opportunity to participate and learn;
- *researcher*, who finds the material needed by the team;
- *encourager*, who reinforces members' contributions;
- *timekeeper*, who monitors time, moves the team along so that they complete the task in the available time and assumes role of any missing team member if there is no wildcard member;
- *recorder*, who takes notes of the team's discussion and prepares a written conclusion;
- *checker*, who makes sure that all team members understand the concepts and the team's conclusions.
- *wildcard*, assumes role of any missing member.

Team roles can be delineated differently and considered instead under more general headings:

- task roles: based on the task the individual will perform within the team;
- maintenance roles: based on communication and ensuring effective teamwork;
- personal roles: assumed normally by students new to team learning.

Some tutors simply share information about team roles with their students and then allow students to choose for themselves how they will proceed. This may occur naturally anyway with more advanced students, for whom the assignment of roles can seem ridiculous and may stifle the normal course of conversation and work. Other tutors begin by assigning team roles and rotating them a couple of times during the initial problems so that students begin to understand the kinds of roles they can assume. Rotating roles can give each student the opportunity to take the lead in a team situation, a role that shy or introverted students sometimes avoid; and it can provide a chance for a dominating student to take a role that involves less talking, thereby creating an opportunity for other students to participate more easily. An assigned role can help students learn how to participate effectively in teams and ultimately can help build effective team processes. In addition, having roles to play encourages interdependence among team members. At some stage in the process, however, assigned roles will start to feel artificial to them and students will begin to not take them seriously, which of course will completely undermine the purpose of the roles. Students at this stage will perform better if they are allowed to fall into roles naturally and tutors should allow students to decide how they will proceed. In addition, some tutors encourage teams to develop a team-learning contract, such as that contained near the end of Chapter 7.

Understanding conflict

While most instances of conflict within a problem-based learning team will probably be unhelpful, conflict is not necessarily a bad thing; it can result in creative confrontation in which new solutions or approaches emerge as a result of the interaction of the conflicting parties. Indeed, many technological breakthroughs have been achieved by that method and in the face of, or perhaps even because of, repeated failures with the existing approaches. However, conflict is not normally associated with creativity; rather, conflict is more likely to be accompanied by hurt, loss and fragmentation of the relationship. Face-to-face communication is the most effective way of understanding what is being communicated since it allows for both verbal and non-verbal exchanges. The trouble is that many of the ways we communicate today ignore the non-verbal signals people give, and even in terrestrial learning teams (as opposed to virtual ones) students may not understand the difference between conflict and assertion. We believe that it is a helpful team-building process to ask students to consider the differences they see between the terms conflict, confrontation, aggression and assertion to enable them to understand the likely impact of each on the team:

- Conflict describes any situation in which two or more people or teams within a community are in opposition. The nature of the opposition may be psychological, spiritual, social or cultural. The conflict may be intra-personal, interpersonal, suppressed, covert or open.

- Confrontation describes a direct encounter in the setting of a conflict; the encounter may be face to face or via telecommunications. Thus it is possible to have a conflict without confrontation, but it is not possible to have a confrontation without conflict.
- Aggression describes conflict behaviour that seeks to harm the other party. It need not be unprovoked, but aggression – by design or by default – seeks to force the wishes of one party on to another at the expense of the former's interests, values or aims.
- Assertion describes behaviour in which one party states clearly their interest, wishes, values or goals. The statement is made so that others might hear and take account of the position and interests of the asserter. However, assertive behaviour also recognizes the rights of the other party and will, therefore, seek to encourage the other party to make a similarly clear statement of their interests, wishes, values and goals. Without this recognition, assertion becomes aggression.

From the above it can be seen that confrontation and assertion may be helpful in the process of conflict resolution. Aggression may lead to resolution through dominance and submission, but it rarely leads to joint problem solving and is likely to contribute to further conflict in the team. Sources of conflict in learning teams generally relate to divergent aims and goals, differing priorities, incompatible strategies and divergent assumptions. Helping students to see the sources and effect of conflict means that they may not necessarily avoid conflict in the team, but they will probably manage conflict better because of their awareness of these issues.

The impact of interactional stances on teams

There is often a sense that the role that staff and students adopt when involved in teamwork differs from other roles at university and in the practice setting. Such roles, and the behaviours that are often assigned to these roles, have been described in detail by such authors as Belbin (1993). While Belbin's role profiles are useful for designing and managing teams whose purpose and identity is defined by a task focus, such a model does not capture the complex interplay of factors occurring for students in the kind of learning teams that are in operation in problem-based contexts. What is needed instead is a set of concepts that together encapsulate the richness and ambiguity of problem-based team learning and interaction. Research into problem-based learning demonstrates that tutors' and students' ability to work and learn effectively within teams is affected by the position they choose to take up within a problem-based leaning team: their interactional stance (Savin-Baden 2000). Interactional stance depicts the way in which a learner interacts with others within a learning situation. It refers to the relationships between students within teams and tutor–student relationships at both an individual and team level. Interactional stance encompasses how students interpret the way they as individuals, and others with whom they learn, construct meaning in relation to one another. The way in which one student may theorize about another student within a team setting reflects his or her interactional stance, as does the way in which a student acts and speaks in interacting with other students. Interactional stance is also a notion that encompasses the means by which students engage with, and attribute meaning to, the processes that occur in teams. It is subsequently through reflection upon these processes that students make sense of their own learning.

Interactional stance: a case example

Nursing students at one UK university found that working and learning in problem-based learning teams had helped them to see the value of shared learning and the advantages of solving problems and difficulties together. In particular, students valued the opportunity problem-based learning offered them, both to discuss with peers problems that had emerged from practice and also to learn to work collaboratively – an opportunity that had not been on offer in other areas of the nursing curriculum.

Emily was a student who had found learning on her own in other areas of the curriculum a difficult task. She had spent the first year of the course writing up lecture notes and revising for examinations. Although she had passed the course thus far, she believed she had forgotten most of what she had learned and merely had six ring binders full of notes to show for her first year of being a nurse. When she went on practice placements she felt she had the basic skills needed for her stage of training, but she constantly felt ill-equipped to transfer the knowledge from exams and essays to the work place. In her second year she began problem-based learning and discovered that learning to solve and manage problems with and through others in the team had helped her to retain the information more effectively than before and to use other people's experiences to understand concepts and practice when she encountered barriers to learning.

This support, which developed throughout teams across the cohort, meant that students were able to spend time reflecting upon their placements and working through difficulties together. By obtaining a number of differing perspectives about how to address a problem, students were able to return to their placement with a number of new strategies and a greater understanding of their experiences. Thus issues, which initially may have appeared complex and irresolvable for an individual, became a team project through which team members facilitated each other in making sense of individual concerns.

The impact of interactional stances on teams

The concept of interactional stance contains four domains and students tend to adopt one of these in the context of the team in which they are learning. Both student–student and tutor–student relationships are affected by the different domains that individuals adopt. Yet students do not just adopt one domain at all times. The way students operate in teams is affected by a number of factors. For example, students' perspectives about what counts as knowledge, their views of themselves as learners and as contributors or not to the team, their prior experience of learning in teams and their concept of the role of the facilitator will all affect the domain that they adopt. The four domains of interactional stance are presented in Figure 8.1.

These four domains can be delineated as follows:

Individualism
Individualism depicts the notion that some students see learning within the team as an activity that is only valuable in terms of what they as an individual can gain from it. These students place little value upon collective learning experiences and are more concerned that they may forgo marks by expending effort sharing tasks and information within the team rather than if they worked alone. Interactional stance as captured within this domain is characterised by the individual placing himself at the centre of the value system.

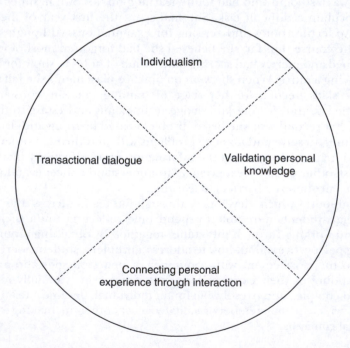

Figure 8.1 Domains within interactional stance

Thus learning within the team is an activity that is only valuable in terms of personal gain for the individual. For example, Phil was a student who had fixed ideas about the method by which the problem should be solved and the way he wanted the feedback report (which was to be assessed) to be produced. Phil found it difficult to accept that other people in his team also had their own ideas and that his idea was not always the best one. He felt disadvantaged by not being in control of the work and invariably offered to be the team member who collated the report so that he could ensure that the team's chances of obtaining the highest marks were maximized. Phil thus used strategies that ensured that he as an individual would gain the best possible marks, even if this meant overruling team opinions and collective values.

Validating personal knowledge

Much of the real learning that occurs through problem-based learning ensues through team interaction, but this is not often rewarded in academic terms. The domain of validating personal knowledge captures the idea that through the experience of being heard within a team and being valued by other team members, individual students learn to value their own knowledge and experience. Students tend to speak of 'making sense', 'connecting', 'seeing things in a new way', all within the context of the team. Thus for many students, learning which occurs in relation to the team process actually holds more meaning than learning which is rewarded through assessment. Rachel, for example, was someone who had discovered that in one problem scenario she was one of the experts in her team in paediatrics because of her prior experience of working in this field. Being an expert helped her to develop confidence and realize the value of her prior experiences both to herself and to the team.

Connecting personal experience through interaction

Students in this domain tend to speak of the way in which learning and reflection within teams enables them to make sense of their own experience as learners. Thus students use teams to make sense of the interrelationship of their problem-solving processes, prior experience and the new material being learned. For example, Bill's prior experience of didactic methods meant he could not understand how he could learn through discussing the problem or how students' differing approaches to problem-solving could possibly produce a cohesive team and an effective answer. Personal reflection, along with reflection and discussion with others, had enabled Bill to explore not only the unresolved set problem, but also his difficulty of being at an impasse in the problem-solving process. Through dialogue with peers he was able to consider how to tackle the given problem and thus integrate that which had been incomprehensible and unfamiliar into his life-world.

Transactional dialogue

In this domain the team serves as an interactive function for the individual. Here dialogue is central to progress in people's lives, since through it values are deconstructed and reconstructed and experiences relived and explored, in order to make sense of roles and relationships. For example, Douglas was a student for whom learning to work in a team was not just about learning how to learn in a team environment, but also learning about democracy, loyalty and effective teamwork. He learned that his focus had to be the achievement of the task with a spirit of cooperation, rather than putting his needs before the achievement of the task. Although in terms of the course he realized that the aim was to solve the given problem, he saw learning in teams in the broader context of offering the opportunity to understand and explore other people's perspectives. Douglas talked about this in terms of 'learning to exist with people' and 'choosing to get on with them'. For him learning with and through others was something that required effort and had to be worked at, and it was only through this that he could hope to understand other people's perspectives. Dialogue offered Douglas the opportunity to explore differing ways of knowing that would ultimately offer him a deeper understanding of the way in which roles and relationships affected his effectiveness as future professional.

Thus interactional stance encompasses how students interpret the way they as individuals and others with whom they learn, construct meaning in relation to one another. Yet the domain students take up reflects not just their own perspectives and motivations, but also their views about the effectiveness of their team, its purpose and the extent to which the team and the facilitator prompt and enhance effective team learning. In order for teams to work effectively, it is important that team members are clear not only about their individual role and perspectives in the team but also the aims and goals of the team as a whole. It is only through such understanding that effective team motivation and commitment can be achieved.

Conclusion

In problem-based learning seminars, student roles dramatically shift not only when they first change to problem-based learning from more traditional approaches but also as they move from being novices to experienced participants in the problem-based learning process. Students begin to share responsibility for their learning and to take some ownership of it, as well as assuming multiple and changing roles within this new context as they face myriad responsibilities. Even though these roles empower students in profound ways, many students are not prepared or inclined to accept them and this creates role anxiety in some cases. However, what is vital for students is that facilitators are also clear about their role. In the next two chapters we explore the role of the facilitator and some ways of helping tutors, when becoming problem-based learning facilitators, to develop and realize their capabilities.

9

The role of tutors

Introduction

There has been considerable discussion about the role of the facilitator in problem-based learning, and in recent years there has been an increase in research in this field. In this chapter we summarize the key areas of literature that deal with many of the questions about the role of tutors. The chapter begins by exploring whether facilitation demands a change in role or just the development of particular skills. However, many tutors struggle to know how to begin the process of facilitation when they first encounter problem-based learning, and therefore we have included a section on useful strategies and issues to consider when learning to facilitate. The final section of the chapter deals with the relative importance of being a content expert and presents recent findings about what actually occurs 'inside' problem-based learning seminars.

Changing roles?

Many people have questioned whether the role of tutors is any different in problem-based learning compared with lecture-based approaches. Although we would argue that it is, we also suggest that much of the role change depends upon the way in which problem-based learning has been implemented within the curriculum. When tutors have designed programmes with problem-based learning as the central curriculum strategy, the effect on roles is likely to be greater than where problem-based learning has just been adopted within one module. Recent research (Savin-Baden 2003) indicated that in programmes where problem-based learning has been adopted wholesale across a curriculum there have been pedagogical challenges and shifts for tutors. Although this was a UK study, the issues raised by tutors, such as feelings of disjunction and loss of power and control, were common in other European countries using problem-based learning in the same way, but this seems not to be the case in universities where much of the problem-based learning utilized is in the form of an instructional design strategy.

For many tutors engaged in problem-based learning the transition from tutor to facilitator demands revising their assumptions about what it means to be a teacher in higher education. The move towards becoming a facilitator invariably demands recognition of a loss of power and control. For many tutors becoming a facilitator is a daunting experience because although they may have taught students through workshops and small group sessions, their role as a facilitator in problem-based learning often requires more of them than in these other forms of teaching. Promoting autonomy in small teams and allowing students to own their own learning experiences involves letting go of decisions about what students should learn, trusting students to acquire knowledge for themselves and accepting that students will learn even if they have not been supplied with a lecture or handout. The conflict for many tutors is in moving from being the controllers and patrollers of knowledge to instead allowing students to manage knowledge for themselves.

Facilitation role or facilitation skills?

There has been much debate about whether facilitation demands particular skills, and Margetson (1994, 1997) believes that facilitation is just good teaching in the sense that it requires the use of abilities that tutors already possess such as probing, questioning, critical reflection, suggesting and where necessary, challenging. However, Margetson's view conflicts with those of Katz (1995) and Wetzel (1996), who argue that new skills need to be learned, a perspective supported by Des Marchais (1993), who argues that different pedagogical expertise is required and that facilitator training needs to be an integral component of changing curricula toward problem-based learning. More recently Oliffe (2000), based on his own experience of becoming a problem-based learning facilitator, argued that facilitation was not a skill commonly used in academic life.

In terms of research into facilitation in problem-based learning, Gijselaers and Schmidt (1990) found that tutor action had a direct causal influence on team tutorials, which in turn influenced students' interest in the subject matter. These findings reflect the complexities involved in the facilitation of problem-based learning. Dolmans *et al.* (1994a) developed a means of assessing tutor performance in problem-based learning teams, but their measurements made no allowance for the inclusion of personal attributes as suggested in earlier work by such authors as Heron (1989) and Jaques (as described in Jaques 2000).

Dolmans's tutor evaluation questionnaire comprised 13 statements concerning tutors' behaviour. Although this instrument was found to be valid and reliable, it seems that it neither accounted for changes in group process nor the need for different types of facilitation at different stages in the programme. A further shortcoming of this study was the lack of definition of what constituted an effective facilitator role. A later study carried out in the same department (Dolmans *et al.* 1994b) argued that tutor evaluation should be embedded in a broader tutors' development programme. The authors argued that such training should include the development of the formal role of the tutor, the stimulation of tutors' dialogue, the design of a tutor-reward system and remedial learning opportunities for tutors. The authors concluded that the study demonstrated that concerted effort being given to a tutor development programme resulted in increasing attention being paid to teaching activities within the medical school.

Research has also explored perceptions of group dynamics (Mpofu *et al.* 1998), the role of the facilitator (Neville 1999), and the perceived effectiveness of tutors. One of the most extensive quantitative studies in this area was undertaken at the University of Maastricht, who have been spearheading work in this area for a number of years. De Grave *et al.* (1998, 1999) focused on developing and testing a tutor intervention profile that sought to determine profiles of effective and less effective tutors. They suggested that the profile distinguishes between tutors who focus students on the acquisition of propositional knowledge (expert knowledge) and those who use process skills to stimulate learning. The findings indicate that tutors who stressed the learning process rather than content acquisition were perceived to be more effective – although, as they point out, the differences found were not statistically significant. What is problematic about many of these studies is that they tend to generalize the behaviour and outcomes of facilitators, rather than exploring the impact of tutors' particular personal and pedagogical stances in the nature and process of facilitation. Furthermore, the notion of learning context and the impact of that context on student learning are rarely seen as variables that need to be taken into account.

However, Gijselaers (1997) examined contextual factors on tutors' behaviours and the effects of departmental affiliation on tutoring. Quantitative analysis of data indicated that overall the level of stability in tutor behaviour, which was examined across different problem-based learning teams, was low, as was the generalizability. However, there still appears to be an assumption that there are specific roles, attributes and ways of being that characterize facilitation that is 'good' or 'better' than others.

Facilitators and students influence one another in a whole variety of ways, such as their views about what counts as knowledge, the interplay of content and process, and the ways in which they do and do not deal with conflict in the team. Facilitators and problem-based learning teams tend to shape and challenge each other, so, while most teams will meet the learning objectives of the programme or module as a minimum, they will do so in different ways because of the team dynamics and the academic positioning of the facilitator. Facilitators have spoken of sitting on their hands, looking out of the window or mentally planning their social life while 'facilitating' a problem-based learning team. Such strategies were designed to prevent them from interfering with and directing the team, but in fact resulted in a good deal of confusion for students who felt that the facilitator did not want to be present.

Getting started as a facilitator

Although there has been considerable research into the facilitator role, there has been relatively little real exploration of what is meant by facilitation, facilitator or the role of the facilitator by either researchers or participants in the research. This confusion is not only seen in the research but also in the way tutors are equipped for implementing problem-based learning. For example, many tutors undergo facilitator training programmes, but as yet there seems to be little distinction made between the different but overlapping roles. One way of engaging with this difficulty would be to argue for role distinctions such as team facilitator, problem-based learning tutor and programme manager. Equipping someone to facilitate a problem-based learning team (a team facilitator) is a task that requires fewer capabilities than the role of facilitating a team while also designing materials and other problem-based learning components of the curriculum (a problem-based learning tutor). A further role might be that of problem-based learning programme manager, who designs the programme and oversees the implementation of problem-based learning but may or may not be a problem-based learning tutor or team facilitator. Although these roles do, to a large extent, overlap, the distinction is important when undertaking research into what might count as effective facilitation.

Heron (1989, 1993) has suggested three modes of facilitation that are useful for helping novice facilitators to consider how they operate. They are as follows:

- *The hierarchical mode*: Here the facilitators direct the learning process and exercise their power over it. Thus they decide (however covertly) the objectives of the team, challenge resistances, manage team feeling and provide structures for learning. In short, the facilitators take responsibility for the learning that takes place.
- *The cooperative mode*: The facilitators share their power over the learning with the team and enable the team to become more self-directed by conferring with them. The facilitators prompt the team members to decide how they are going to learn and to manage confrontation. Although the facilitators share their own views, they are not seen as final but as one view among many.
- *The autonomous mode*: The facilitators respect the total autonomy of the team; the facilitators do not do things for them or with them but give them the space and freedom to do things their own way. Without guidance, reminders or assistance, the team evolves its learning and structure, finds its own ways to manage conflict and gives meaning to personal and team learning. The facilitator's role is that of creating conditions in which students can exercise self-determination in their learning.

The modes are not designed to be discrete or hierarchical and do, to some extent overlap with one another. These are useful guides, particularly when coupled with the further descriptions that Heron has added, but there are also some rather obvious and helpful issues that need to be considered when learning to be a facilitator, which include:

1   *Acknowledging and using prior experience.* Many tutors feel that becoming a facilitator seems to be such a different role when they first begin that often they forget to draw on their prior experience. It is important to draw on earlier experiences. For example, one approach might be to reflect on the experience of being supervised in a research project. Often the supervisor guides the students in the early stages of the project, but toward the end the students may overtake their knowledge base. Another option might be to imagine the facilitator role as being that of a non-directive counsellor who uses reflection and questioning rather than direction.

2   *Recognizing that being a facilitator means also being a learner.* This might mean learning to develop the capabilities of a facilitator and possibly also learning new knowledge with and through the students. The process of becoming a facilitator also demands developing and understanding the way in which facilitator and team influence one another in the learning process.

3   *Ensuring that the team's concerns are heard.* Active listening skills are a prerequisite to good communication and are one of the most effective tools for resolving conflicts. An ability to listen to the team's concerns and problems sets the foundation for a positive relationship that encourages honesty, trust and understanding.

4   *Being responsive to team concerns.* Facilitators who are able to respond quickly and flexibly are better positioned to respond effectively to issues that arise in the team. Too often the structural arrangements of the timetable are so complex that teams and facilitators are inhibited in their decision-making and denied the autonomy and flexibility that is needed in problem-based learning.

5   *Appreciating shared risk.* In order to enjoy the benefits of an alliance, teams should first be prepared to share any associated risks as well as the benefits. These risks are not simply pedagogical but are personal too in terms of the challenges problem-based learning can bring to peoples' lives and prior experiences of learning.

Stimulating discussion and enabling the team

There is often an assumption that stimulating discussion necessarily means some kind of verbal intervention by the facilitator. However, when a team is first presented with the problem, it is important that they begin the discussion themselves with little, if any intervention from the tutor. Managing silence can be difficult but Wilkie's study (Wilkie 2002) found that tutors' perception of team silence was considerably longer than the actual silence recorded on the audio recorder. However, it is often the case that students are talkative in the student common room and in the corridors but not in the seminar, and after the initial remarks made about the problem, the conversation in the classroom can remain difficult and stilted. There are a number of perspectives about the extent to which a facilitator should intervene in a problem-based learning seminar, which to some extent relates to the way in which the facilitator role is seen, initially. For example, Boud and Feletti (1997) have suggested the role of the facilitator is that of a planner, evaluator, resource person and an instrument of social action and change. Thus here one would assume that intervention would be considerable because of the focus on action and change. However, Brookfield (1985), although not speaking directly to the world of problem-based learning, sees facilitation as a form of transactional dialogue, so here the focus would be on a kind of facilitation that promotes critical reflection and evaluation of students' ideas and experiences. Stimulating discussion can be prompted by some of the following strategies.

Non-verbal strategies

1   *Scanning the members*. In problem-based learning seminars, novice students tend to refer questions and information directly to the facilitator. Although it may be difficult (and may seem rude), it is important to glance around the team, thus giving the students the impression that the information and questions are to be shared.
2   *Using gestures*. Gestures can be used very effectively for signalling to team members without interrupting the flow of the discussion too much. For example, nodding or leaning towards a student who wants to speak or using a hand signal to stop someone talking can be very effective. It is important not to give negative messages through gestures, so it is best to avoid gestures such as rolling your eyes or looking out of the window when you do not agree. If you need to intervene because there are shortcomings in the information given, it is better to use an open question such as, 'How does that relate to what Ruth said earlier?'
3   *Picking up cues*. Watching students in the team and picking up cues, such as restlessness, a puzzled frown or a smile can give a good indication of the climate of the team and can help us to know if and when to intervene.

Verbal strategies

1   *Asking questions*. It is important to remember that in the context of problem-based learning, questions should be used to help students to reach a greater level of understanding of the issues under consideration and to analyse the problem presented in depth. It is often a challenge for facilitators to use questions for the right purpose when they are new to problem-based learning; questions should not be used as a controlling mechanism (however covert), and thus open and reflective questions are more appropriate than closed or leading ones.
2   *Supporting and valuing*. Creating an atmosphere of trust and openness

where students can share ideas without fear of being ridiculed is vital to develop and sustain group dynamics. This component of building problem-based learning teams is often lost amid the focus on tasks and assessment, but it is important that the tutor does not constantly correct students. Sometimes a student would like to ask questions but would feel unintelligent and awkward in doing so; if the tutor suspects this and is able to anticipate the questions, she should feel free to ask the questions instead.

3   *Summarizing.* It may sometimes be useful to summarize the position you feel the team has reached in order to help them to move on, or as a means of checking group progress. However, summarizing should not be judgemental, but rather as impartial as possible, stating the group progress and ensuring the team is happy with the summary you offered.

4   *Returning and deflecting questions.* In problem-based learning students often ask the facilitator direct questions. It is important to turn such questions back so that students take responsibility for finding out the information for themselves. Responses such as, 'Well, what do you think? What do other people think?' are useful here.

5   *Suggesting alternatives.* There are some instances when a team either comes to a standstill, unable to decide which way to move next, or opts for a narrow track that means its members will have to do considerable work later to make up for this approach. Sometimes, when students are new to problem-based learning, it is helpful to suggest other avenues such as: 'What do you think about the time you have spent working on that? Perhaps we should look at x now?'

6   *Monitoring progress.* Ideally monitoring the progress of the group is something that should be done by team members themselves, but it is often useful to summarize progress for the team at the end of sessions. This indicates both to them and to you as facilitator how you see the progress of the team.

7   *Reflecting back.* Reflecting back is the process of checking what was said, such as, 'What I heard you say was . . .' When reflecting back it is important to comment accurately rather than give an interpretation about what was said. Further, it is important not to imply that there was an assumption implicit in what was said. Reflecting back is not about offering negative criticism but seeking understanding and clarification of what is occurring, and therefore the facilitator should not impose her view on the situation.

8   *Using reflection.* Reflection is still quite under utilized in problem-based learning teams (Savin-Baden 2003). Reflection is useful as it helps the team to consider both the content and process of the team. This process can be encouraged by the facilitator asking students to respond individually to some reflective question agreed in advance with the team, by asking each team member to offer a reflection at the beginning or end of a session, or by asking students to write a reflective piece about their experience to date that they later share with the rest of their team.

Giving feedback

Facilitators should give feedback to the team, although we have found that this is a controversial issue for some tutors. Some tutors feel that students become over-reliant on them if they give feedback, which prevents the team from developing autonomy in learning. However, feedback is not just about commenting on what was presented, it is also about team process and progress, the interrelationship of the students and facilitator, and the overall group cohesion. Feedback needs to be clear, positive and specific. For example, facilitators should avoid vague and general comments that do not help students such as, 'That went well', or 'You all seem to be doing okay.' It is much better to offer a comment that gives the team or the student some clear feedback that will enable change to take place, for example, 'I think you used PowerPoint very effectively to help the team learn this complex topic, but perhaps next time you could use 10 slides instead of 60, so that you are able to keep within the available time.' In this example the feedback is 'owned'. Instead of saying, 'It might be useful if . . .' it is better to own the statement, 'I feel . . . I think . . .' because it shows that as a facilitator you are taking responsibility for the feedback you are giving.

Facilitator responsibility

Being a responsible facilitator is an area that is debated with great heat and tension. Much of what is executed depends upon the subject area or discipline, but the following points may help some tutors to consider what might count as tutor responsibility while working and learning in a team:

• help students understand informed consent;
• create a forum for students to discuss the ethics involved in teamwork;
• discuss the role and responsibility of the facilitator in the team. Present research that shows facilitator and student development changes, depending on the context and the experience of both;
• design materials to discourage plagiarism, and change these regularly;
• use assessment approaches that reduce plagiarism.

Few problem-based learning teams, particularly in undergraduate education are voluntary; rather problem-based teamwork is a condition of the course. In other approaches, such as action learning, voluntarily joining and remaining a member of an action learning set is founded on the values held by the set (McGill and Beaty 2001). This kind of conditional membership in problem-based learning teams means that values about joining and being committed do not apply in the same way as action learning sets. It may be possible to develop a number of codes or principles to which students comply, but it must be recognized that such codes cannot govern behaviour but only help to guide. For example, the principles of autonomy, non-maleficence and beneficence, and informed consent could be sound starting points for helping a team to develop an ethical framework in which to learn.

Expert and non-expert tutors

Numerous papers and discussions have considered whether tutors need to be content experts when facilitating problem-based learning. Barrows (1988) has argued that problem-based learning facilitators need to be both content experts and skilled tutors. Yet a study undertaken by Kaufman and Holmes (1998) discovered that content experts found it more difficult to maintain a facilitator role than non-experts.

Research at Maastricht has shown that students guided by content experts achieved more than those guided by non-experts (Schmidt 1994). Schmidt and Moust (2000b) argue that comparing expert tutors to non-expert ones along with comparing tutors to student tutors is inconclusive. However, they offer a theory of tutor performance, termed cognitive congruence, which is 'a tutor's ability to understand and to express him or herself at the students' level of knowledge . . . In addition cognitive congruence assumes sensitivity of the tutor concerning the difficulties that students may come across while dealing with a problem or with the subject matter relevant to the problem' (p. 43). Schmidt and Moust tested this theory and found that both social congruence and expertise were important factors in being an effective tutor. Thus they argue that being an effective facilitator of problem-based learning demands three interrelated qualities, namely a knowledge base relevant to the problem being studied, being involved with the students in an authentic way, and being able to communicate with the students at their level of understanding.

Neville (1999) reviewed the role of the tutor in problem-based learning and suggested that novice students with little experience of the approach would probably benefit from directive tutors who were knowledge experts. He argued that such tutors would help students to construct a foundation on which to build their learning. In contrast, he suggested that students more experienced in the approach required less direction as they progressed, because they became increasingly self-sufficient. What is important about Neville's examination of the issues relating to problem-based facilitation is his acknowledgement that different situations require different tutor behaviour in order to facilitate student learning, a finding supported by a recent study by Wilkie (2002).

What actually happens in a problem-based learning seminar?

The issue of what actually occurs 'inside' a problem-based learning seminar is a topic of much discussion for those involved in using this approach. Students have suggested that changing the facilitator every six weeks (or less) is detrimental to their learning and meant that they constantly had to discuss group dynamics, sometimes to the cost of in-depth learning (Savin-Baden 1996). The exploration of the dynamics and process in problem-based seminars is of growing research interest. For example, Virtanen *et al.* (1999) examined medical students' written accounts of successful and unsuccessful problem-based learning seminars. Overall their findings suggest that successful sessions rely on a balanced discussion between team members, pre-seminar preparation by the team, and some, but not too much, intervention by the facilitator. Lack of interest in the seminar by team members and facilitators, as well as passive students and dominant tutors result in unsuccessful sessions.

A study by Curet and Mennin (2003) evaluated the affect of short-term (3–5 weeks) and long-term tutors (6–10 weeks) on students' performance and the quality of the seminars. Although students' performance was not affected by long-term or short-term tutors, they did find that long-term tutors were ranked higher by students with regard to the quality of the tutorial process. It is arguable as to whether a 6–10 week time period could be described as long term in the context of many established problem-based learning pro-grammes where students stay in the same team for six months or even a year. What is problematic about these and earlier studies (for example, Wilkerson *et al.* 1991; Savin-Baden 1996; Koschmann *et al.* 1997) is that tutors and students were not tracked over time, and while the studies present useful snap-shots, they do not explore changes in time and in the experience of both facilitator and team. However Wilkie's study did do this (Wilkie 2002). She examined the strategies adopted by new facilitators in a problem-based learn-ing nursing programme and followed their progress for a two-year period. By interviewing tutors, recording their seminars and interviewing students, she gained a complex perspective of facilitator change and behaviour over time.

The directive conventionalist approach

In the directive conventionalist approach, learning was content-focused and under the direction of the facilitator. Students were encouraged to seek out and learn facts. Aspects of problem-based learning, such as learning skills or promotion of critical thinking, were of less importance than factual content. The characteristic feature of the directive conventionalist approach was the use of convergent, directive questions to elicit content. The approach was associated predominantly with novice facilitators who may have selected it for reasons of familiarity with a lecturer role and feeling in control.

The liberating supporter approach

Facilitators who adopted the liberating supporter approach made minimal interventions in problem-based learning seminars. Within the limits of the problem, the students were free to decide on their own learning, in terms of both the content and learning method. Although there was some emphasis on encouraging students to acquire self-directed learning skills, the overall purpose of the learning was content acquisition rather than learning processes in their own right. This approach was adopted least often. It was the approach which most facilitators, at least in their initial experience of problem-based learning, perceived to epitomize problem-based learning facilitation.

The nurturing socializer approach

The nurturing socializer approach was student-centred, nurturing and supportive. Both facilitators and students made extensive use of narrative. The approach was supportive with facilitators believing that students had to feel valued so that in turn they were able to value and care for patients.

The pragmatic enabler approach

The pragmatic enabler approach developed over time with increased exposure of facilitators to problem-based learning. It was not fully identifiable until the third cycle of the study when it had become the most common approach. The pragmatic enabler approach emphasized learning processes rather than content acquisition. Facilitators related to the requirement to produce qualified practitioners. To enable students to achieve their maximum potential, facilitators required a flexible approach, which was time and context dependent and responsive to the needs of a diverse range of students.

Wilkie found that although every facilitator had a unique style of facilitation, these four approaches were most evident, while being neither fixed nor hierarchical. Instead they were time and context bound. Furthermore, she also defined six further elements (content eliciting, process interventions, engagement, frame factors, narrative and evaluation) that influenced each approach, and despite all of the elements being present in each of the four approaches, they were used to varying degrees and in different ways in each approach.

Conclusion

Being and becoming a facilitator in problem-based learning continues to be an area that provokes much discussion and argument. What is important is that those facilitating such seminars are committed to taking up the role and are not there under protest or disinterest. Being told to take up such a role is likely to be detrimental to student learning and to threaten the longevity of the use of problem-based learning in that particular course or programme. In this chapter we have explored the theory and practice of the facilitator role. Next we turn to ways of equipping tutors to be facilitators in problem-based learning curricula.

10

Staff support and development

Introduction

To date, relatively little has been written about educational development for problem-based learning. Yet there has been a growing debate about the place, position and role of academic and tutor development in higher education in general. Within the problem-based community, it is evident that there are widely-held views about the kinds of development that should be undertaken in order to equip, develop and support tutors in becoming facilitators. This chapter engages with these debates, beginning by exploring current practice and then arguing that tutor development for problem-based learning should start by helping tutors to understand the ways in which they have positioned themselves within higher education. It then explores models of educational development and discusses the challenges of implementing innovation. The final section of the chapter suggests ways of implementing educational development as an integral part of a long-term strategy to support problem-based learning.

Tutor development practices

Many scholars now perceive the area of tutor development to be key to the success of problem-based learning (Nayer 1995). The number of tutor development workshops documented in recent years demonstrates this fact (for example Almy et al. 1992; Holmes and Kaufman 1994; Little 1997; Wilkerson and Hundert 1997; Musal et al. 2002; Zimitat and Miflin 2003). However, few studies have documented the processes and outcomes of tutor development and progress, or evaluated the success of tutor training or indeed tutor perspectives. The role, satisfaction, effectiveness and training of tutors in problem-based learning programmes is still an under-researched area, and literature that is currently available, in general, only documents accounts of tutor development programmes (for example, Del Mar 1997;

Kippers *et al.* 1997; Ryan 1997). What has tended to happen is that general principles of tutor and educational development have been adapted to equip tutors for problem-based learning by consultants who, while well versed in educational development, have never actually implemented problem-based learning themselves, nor designed a problem-based curriculum. Alternatively, tutors wanting to implement problem-based learning read a considerable amount of literature and then attend a generic tutor development workshop on problem-based learning at one of the centres of excellence such as the University of Maastricht, The Netherlands; University of Delaware, USA, or McMaster University, Canada.

All of these strategies may equip tutors to implement problem-based learning, but a number of difficulties exist with them. The first is that using generic tutor development consultants to advise on the implementation of problem-based learning can be very risky if those consultants have never used the approach. They will seldom be aware of some of the stumbling blocks that tutors can experience or of some of the common mistakes that can be made when designing problem-based curricula. Second, attending three-day workshops at one of the centres of excellence, while being informative, is invariably insensitive to cultural and disciplinary differences. This can leave the tutor with the view that they have to do it the 'McMaster way' or adopt 'the seven-step model' developed by Maastricht, instead of developing a model that will suit their university and disciplinary culture and fit with the needs of their programme.

Thus in order to implement problem-based learning in a way that promotes sound educational development, it is important to plan its introduction into the curriculum. It is best introduced one or two years before the whole curriculum is changed. This will allow sufficient time to decide on the kind of programme that is to be designed and to prepare tutors adequately for the introduction of this new approach. However, in practice, time constraints rarely provide the opportunity for such a long-range approach.

Many tutors wanting to introduce problem-based learning begin by making a few modules problem-based, and then having become used to the approach, spend time redesigning the curriculum as a whole. This incremental approach works effectively and also helps tutors to adjust over a period of time. However, few of the development programmes discussed in the literature deal with the challenges that tutors face or the nature or type of development on offer.

Beginning with ourselves

The proliferation of courses and curricula that have adopted problem-based learning has meant that there has been a greater demand for tutor development workshops, consultancy, mentoring and guidance than in former years. For many tutors, the notion of 'being equipped' or 'developed' is seen as deeply problematic, and for some it is even seen as an insult to their capabilities as a tutor. Indeed Webb has argued:

> When initiatives to introduce problem-based learning, or better small-group discussion, or better lecturing come to be written up, the human side of a staff development relationship seldom comes through. We have theories of learning and teaching, practical techniques and prescriptions, but seldom any insight into the *personal* nature of the process from which the abstractions are drawn.
>
> (Webb 1996: 36)

Yet we suggest that equipping tutors for engaging with problem-based learning is an important activity because it involves more than just learning the nuts and bolts of how to implement it. Instead it requires that we examine our own views about the nature of teaching and learning, knowledge and cognition. Problem-based learning, because it is an approach through which we can encourage students to own their learning experiences and develop independence in inquiry, forces us to consider our ontological positions as tutors and learners. Thus helping tutors to explore their views of themselves as teachers is an important part of the process of becoming a facilitator. This can be undertaken by using case studies of teaching (for example, Schwartz and Webb 1993) because it helps tutors to see that what they may see as a straightforward way of teaching can be hugely problematic for someone else. Tutors also often forget the extent to which their political views, feminist perspectives, culture and class views influence not only the way in which they teach but also the things they encourage and discourage in a learning context. Equipping tutors for problem-based learning does not only begin with discussions about what counts as problem-based learning, or arguments about the relative merits of different ways of implementation, but also the business of examining our own personal, pedagogical and interactional stances towards learners and learning.

Theories and models of academic development

In recent years there have been discussions about whether the process of equipping tutors is a process of tutor, educational or academic development (Webb 1996; Eggins and Macdonald 2003). These debates have highlighted the importance of whether it is the development of teaching and learning within the institution we are debating, the individual tutor's ability to be equipped to teach better – to be developed, or whether it is something else. Often the terms 'staff development' and 'educational development' are used interchangeably, but there is a growing trend to use the term 'academic development' as a catch-all. Much of the literature on problem-based learning tends towards staff development that focuses upon equipping tutors with skills to implement the approach through training workshops that offer hints and tips. However, we believe this approach demands appropriate educational development that works with tutors to help them manage their educational challenges and problems (following Baume and Baume 1994). It is in the context of this argument that we suggest six approaches to educational development that are in operation with regard to problem-based learning. These approaches are based on the work of Boud and McDonald (1981) and the research of Land (2003).

Professional service model

In this model an external consultant is employed to guide tutors in the design and implementation of problem-based learning within the programme. The consultant usually runs a series of workshops on the nature of problem-based learning and its design features and helps the process of implementation over a period of time. Universities or disciplines with substantial funding to sustain this model, particularly those who see the adoption of problem-based learning as an important and long-term approach to teaching, adopt this tactic.

Managerial model

In this approach the university management has decided to adopt problem-based learning as a major component of the institutional learning strategy. Institutional goals drive the focus of the educational development and the use (or not) of an external expert. Thus the change to problem-based learning is managed in a directive fashion, and the result is often the use of diverse and sometimes conflicting models of problem-based learning within different courses and programmes, which may result in confusion for both tutors and students.

Entrepreneurial model

In this model, problem-based learning is often implemented as a result of monies gained for innovation, or is seen as a project that will later gain money and status for the individuals involved in its introduction. The focus on educational development here is equipping tutors to implement problem-based learning quickly for political reasons and then encouraging them to be evangelists for the approach. This kind of educational development results in status for all those involved and tends to be utilized as a means of career development. Educational development here becomes tutor development, and generic workshops, run to equip people to introduce problem-based learning, are invariably done 'infotainment' style: a liberal mix of information and entertainment (Ritzer 1996).

Romantic model

This approach is about developing tutors involved in problem-based learning, not just in relation to the implementation of the approach, but with a concern for their personal development and inner growth as a central component of the strategy. Such an approach stands in direct conflict with the managerial and entrepreneurial approaches, and workshops are invariably run in a Rogerian style with tutor concerns and reflections as the central focus of learning for all those involved. This kind of educational development tends to be run in-house by those keen to develop problem-based learning within the university. The educational developers have humanistic beliefs about the nature of educational development and see problem-based learning as a means of promoting liberal education despite the global trends towards consumerism and commerce-driven education.

Counselling model

In this model, an external consultant or an expert in problem-based learning from another discipline in the same university, provides opportunities for tutors to explore the difficulties they are experiencing with the implementation or long-term sustainability of problem-based learning. Those who have implemented problem-based learning with little or no external help, and who then seek guidance when difficulties arise, often use this model.

Professional competence model

This model is commonly adopted when several tutors have attended courses or conferences on problem-based learning and have been experimenting with the approach for a year or so. Educational development here is seen as bringing these tutors up to a baseline of competence in using the approach. Such workshops are often undertaken as generic master classes, designed to help people to learn from one another and also to get extra tips from the expert who has been brought in to run the sessions. In such workshops tutors bring in videos of themselves in action or present problem scenarios that they have developed, so that colleagues and the workshop facilitator can critique them. This kind of educational development is designed to build skills, competence and confidence.

Discipline-based or generic educational development?

Generic workshops for introducing tutors to problem-based learning still tend to be the dominant model in use globally. For example, what often occurs is the employment of a problem-based learning consultant to run a one- or possibly two-day workshop within a university to help their tutors to examine the ways it might be implemented within their university. This is a useful approach to help multiple tutors from different fields to establish a common vocabulary and to develop a common conception of problem-based learning. However, it is also important to engage with disciplinary differences, and this is becoming a growing trend in the UK with the development of national subject centres. Our belief that on-going educational development should predominantly be located within the disciplines stems from our experience that generic workshops do not offer tutors the opportunity to engage with the complexities of what it means to teach and manage knowledge in ways that discipline-based workshops do. This is because most tutors' allegiance is to their discipline and many of those disciplines adopt distinctive forms of teaching and particular conceptions of knowledge. Thus problem-based learning needs to be translated into the culture of that discipline and adapted to meet its values and ideologies. However, we recognize, as Delanty suggests, that 'Disciplinary boundaries are becoming blurred as multidisciplinarity becomes the norm and as the new phenomenon of "postdisciplinarity" takes over (Turner 1999)' (Delanty 2001: 3). Thus spaces need to be provided for postdisciplinary tutor development as well.

The challenges of tutor development

We suggest that one of the main difficulties in developing problem-based learning within a curriculum is the way in which tutor development is carried out. This kind of development can be an area of great sensitivity to tutors who have been experts in their disciplines and subjects for many years. Many tutors find changing their roles to be a complex and difficult process. The analogy of crossing the chasm (Moore 1999, following Rogers 1962) is a useful way of engaging with many of the issues related to implementing an innovation such as problem-based learning and dealing with tutor reactions to this new approach. Moore's work relates to the development and adoption of technology within companies. He argued that there is a chasm between two distinct marketplaces: an early market that tends to be dominated by those keen to take it on board (early adopters), along with insiders who quickly see the benefit of the new development. The second marketplace is characterized by a range of people who ultimately want the benefits of the new technology but are slower to take it up and more cynical about its possibilities. What tends to occur is the emergence of a chasm between those in the early market and those in the later mainstream market. We suggest that crossing this chasm is an important focus for those involved in any innovation. For those tutors who have been involved in developing problem-based learning curricula, this image, as shown in Figure 10.1, is often helpful in enabling them to understand the struggles they encounter when implementing this challenging approach. This is because Moore's image

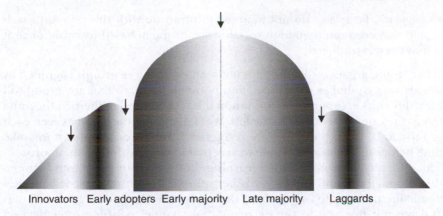

Innovators   Early adopters   Early majority   Late majority   Laggards

Figure 10.1   The adoption life cycle

helps us to see why there are problems not only with the implementation of technology but also with any innovation that affects people's lives and ways of seeing the world.

Moore refers to products (in this case problem-based learning) as discontinuous innovations that require people to change behaviour or to modify other areas within the organization. The original research that led to this model of the technology adoption life cycle related to the purchasing of new strains of seed potatoes among American farmers (Rogers 1962). In this original adoption and diffusion model Rogers argued that people tend to respond to innovation in five particular ways. We have adapted these to refer to educational innovation and the kinds of reactions to problem-based learning that tutors may have when it is introduced:

- *Innovators, the enthusiasts* pursue both the idea and the implementation of problem-based learning aggressively. Innovation and change is central to their focus and *raison d'être* in higher education and problem-based learning is often their latest obsession.
- *Early adopters, the visionaries* are like innovators in that they get involved in a project such as problem-based learning early on, once the decision to implement it has been made. They rely on their own intuition about the benefits of the approach and are central to the implementation of such a development, because they find it easy to imagine the benefits of the approach.
- *Early majority, the pragmatists* are a group who share some of the early adopters' ability to see the benefits of the approach but they tend to be immensely practical, are aware of the dangers of passing fads and so are content to wait to see if it is likely to be successful before they commit themselves to this approach.
- *Late majority, the conservatives* share the same concerns as the early majority but they are not comfortable with the introduction of new approaches and so they will wait until it has become an established mode of practice.

- *Laggards, the sceptics* do not want anything to do with this new approach and will even often attempt to sabotage problem-based learning once it has been introduced.

What Moore argues is that the gaps between each pair of groups (signified by the arrows) symbolize the dissociation between them, so that any group will have difficulty accepting the innovation if it is presented to them in the same way as the one immediately to the left. We suggest that the gaps between each group can be managed if they are recognized, and we accept that it will take time before most tutors feel able to accept and work with the new approach. The difficulty in problem-based learning, however, is in the chasm between the late majority and the laggards because it is often disregarded. In academic life it is easy to forget about those who are always doing other things and are not involved in the departmental change towards problem-based learning, so we disregard them. While it is important not to force the sceptics into becoming facilitators, it is vital that they are not left alone to sabotage the process. So we offer a few strategies to consider when implementing problem-based learning that will inform the possibilities for educational development in your institution:

Strategies for crossing and managing the gaps and the chasm

1   Use different types of educational development approaches for each group.
2   Demonstrate to the early adopters how problem-based learning has worked effectively in other disciplines and universities.
3   Once the early majority have become familiar with problem-based learning, find ways of making it easier for the late majority to adopt. For example, provide opportunities for them to watch it in action, and/or provide a buddy system for new facilitators.
4   Accept that the late majority will take time to adjust and that many will need both considerable time and research evidence. Give them time to think, read and question.
5   Do not take criticism personally; see all criticism as part of the process of progress.
6   Do not force the laggards to become involved, but instead negotiate with them as to what they are prepared to do without feeling compromised. This might include providing you with supporting lectures or laboratory sessions.
7   Be realistic about what is possible within your department and ensure you have allowed enough time for implementation. Many people try to implement problem-based learning too quickly and so face resistance from the early majority, which tends to be one of the fastest ways to fail at the outset.

8   Accept that laggards may take time to get involved, but that ultimately if
     they do not do so, they pose a threat to the long-term sustainability of
     your problem-based learning.

Implementing tutor development programmes: the realities

Using the model of Moore's chasm, it is therefore possible to see that introducing problem-based learning and equipping tutors is a complex and often
contested business. However, we suggest that commencing implementation
with a two- to three-day workshop is advisable. In such a workshop you will
probably have a few innovators but in the main early adopters, whom the
innovators may irritate, but who will want to explore the possibilities of the
approach. Such a workshop can be undertaken over two or three consecutive
days or one day a week over two or three weeks. There should be no more
than twenty participants, and tutors should be committed to attending all of
the days. This is because spending time as a group working through the
issues helps tutors to grapple with them in depth, and these tutors subsequently become much clearer about the issues relating to the implementation of problem-based learning. A longer period also helps tutors to deal
with any disjunction they experience regarding problem-based learning and
gives them the opportunity to share their concerns. In the current climate of
higher education, where student numbers are high and tutor time is very
limited for learning about new approaches, it could be argued that this is a
very expensive form of educational development. However, programmes
where problem-based learning have been implemented successfully and
maintained over time have invariably been the ones that, from the outset,
have put time and funding into equipping tutors to implement it. A detailed
example of initial preparation of facilitators is presented in Murray and
Savin-Baden (2000).

Long-term development programmes

It is often the case that once a programme of educational development has
been undertaken, tutors are then expected to implement the curriculum
with little ongoing support. Yet for many tutors the implementation of the
programme and the provision of support while they become familiar with
the approach are as important as the initial workshops. Recent research
(Savin-Baden 2003; Wilkie 2002) has shown that tutor roles as facilitators
evolve over time, and that many have required support as they make the shift
away from more didactic approaches, characterized by giving clear directions
to students about what and how to learn and providing short talks in the
problem-based learning sessions, towards the adoption of dialogic facilitation. What we mean by dialogic facilitation is a position whereby the facilitator

is able to be part of a team debate without imposing his own agenda and can promote learning through dialogue without directing the students about what should be learned. Wilkie's research has demonstrated that facilitators do change and adapt their role over a period of time and that their ability to become less controlling and directing is related to their pedagogical beliefs. Wilkie's research seems to indicate that ongoing support is required in order to help facilitators to adapt their role over time, as the students become more familiar with problem-based learning and more sophisticated as learners.

Action learning sets

Action learning is a useful approach for helping tutors involved in problem-based learning to discuss the challenges they are experiencing and review problem scenarios and the evolution of the curriculum. In practice, the facilitators meet in groups of six to eight, to deal with the issues relating to facilitation and the challenges that this has brought to them personally and pedagogically. These sets are ideal for both providing support and resolving issues, since individuals help each other to move forward with their concerns. Furthermore, the set is more than a support group because tutors learn about themselves, each other and problem-based learning through a continuous process of reflecting and acting on an individual's problem. However, it is important that the sets are formalized and that they meet on a regular basis to undertake action that will deal with or resolve problems.

Coaching and mentoring

There is increasing interest in the use of coaching and mentoring in many areas of higher education including the problem-based learning community. It often begins when a tutor is attempting to implement problem-based learning single-handed and she looks to someone with greater experience for advice. In our experience, this is often undertaken as an informal process but we believe that formal mentoring is an important support mechanism for tutors involved in problem-based learning.

There are many definitions of coaching; some people look at it from an academic point of view, many from a sporting perspective. The principle feature of coaching from both perspectives is that it is learner-centred; the coach does not tell the individual what to learn but provides him or her with experiences that will lead the individual to find those things out for themselves. Coaching is about unlocking people's potential to maximize their own performance. It is helping them to learn rather than teaching them so that their awareness is raised about what is happening around them. It is also about encouraging full responsibility for thoughts, actions and outcomes. When we accept, choose and take responsibility for our thoughts and actions, our commitment to them rises and so does our performance. Coaching is often used at work for the following reasons:

- motivating tutors;
- delegating;
- problem solving;
- relationship issue;
- team building;

- appraisal;
- assessment;
- task performance;
- planning and reviewing;
- tutor development.

Coaching is not merely a technique to be used by line managers and applied when faced with performance issues. It is a way of managing, a way of treating people and a way of thinking. Furthermore, most of the essential skills and behaviours for coaching are concerned with helping the coachee become aware of what is going on, for example by use of

- open questioning technique;
- active listening;
- clarifying goals and commitment;
- non-judgemental comment;
- silence to create space for reflection.

In some texts mentoring and coaching are used synonymously, but we suggest that although they have similar traits, there are some important differences. Mentoring is usually done by a colleague or peer rather than a line manager and focuses on personal change rather than organizational or task goals, or outcomes. The individual usually chooses a mentor and the relationship between mentor and mentee is one of equality – although the mentor may offer advice. In the context of problem-based learning, a mentor would be someone with whom you shared the challenges of working with the approach and who would support you in making the changes appropriate to facilitate your own learning and the learning of others. Some of the differences between coaching and mentoring are illustrated in Table 10.2.

Table 10.2 A comparison of coaching and mentoring

Feature	Coaching	Mentoring
Focus on	Skill	Personal development
Time scale	Short to medium	Medium to long
Basis of approach	Goal oriented	Transformation
Style	Expert goal setter	Reflective enabler
Relationship	Superior	Equal
Motivation	Improving performance	Guiding and modelling
Structure	Formal	Informal
Learning approach	Behavioural or cognitive	Developmental or critical awareness
Perception of role	Expert task setter	Orchestrator of opportunities
Outcomes	Measurable change	Reported shifts

Master classes
After tutors have undertaken educational development and then implemented problem-based learning, many feel that support groups are helpful
for resolving issues, but neither help them to further develop their capabilities as facilitators nor enable them to design more complex materials for
problem-based learning. What has been helpful for many tutors a year or so
after the implementation of problem-based learning is a series of master
classes. These are interactive workshop sessions on topics suggested by the
tutors but facilitated by an external expert. Topics for this may include
reviewing the assessment process, developing complex trigger materials and
examining tutors' stances in the facilitation process. These master classes are
designed to be informative, help tutors examine the latest research on the
given topic and offer tutors an opportunity to engage in-depth with an issue.
However, such classes do need to be located within a long-term development
strategy or to be part of action learning sets, otherwise they will just be seen
by both tutors and the institution as quick top-up sessions rather than part of
a sound overall educational development strategy.

Conclusion

The current shift towards problem-based learning within higher education
means that educational development needs to be a central component in
any problem-based learning implementation strategy. Such a strategy needs
to take account of not only institutional and tutor support but also the type
of scheme of educational development to be adopted. As we have seen, there
are a number of approaches to educational development that need to be
considered, and it is important that both short and long-term strategies are
planned. However, the pedagogical positions of the tutors involved also
needs to be considered in terms of their beliefs about learning, the values
they hold about student autonomy and their reactions to innovation and
change.

11

Assessing problem-based learning

Introduction

Issues about the impact of assessment on student learning, both on traditional and problem-based curricula, have been the subject of much debate and education research. The whole area of assessment is fraught with difficulties. At one level there are assumptions that if there is a fit between learning methods, module objectives and assessment then there will be few problems. At another, it can be argued that it is impossible to assess students without falling into hegemonic practices. This chapter explores the role and purpose of assessment in higher education and examines issues about assessment that are particular to problem-based learning. Although issues of assessment and evaluation are often interlinked we discuss programme evaluation in depth in Chapter 13.

Definitions of assessment

Interest in assessment by tutors has grown in popularity in the last few decades, as increased calls for accountability have prompted educators to offer more proof that what they are doing is successful. However, assessment has not been an easy term to define, and its definition has gone through several iterations. A widely accepted definition of assessment is as follows:

> Assessment is an ongoing process aimed at understanding and improving student learning. It involves making our expectations explicit and public; setting appropriate criteria and high standards for learning quality; systematically gathering, analysing and interpreting evidence to determine how well performance matches those expectations and standards; and using the resulting information to document, explain and improve performance. When it is embedded effectively within larger institutional systems, assessment can help us focus our collective

attention, examine our assumptions and create a shared academic culture dedicated to assuring and improving the quality of higher education.

(Angelo 1995: 7)

There are some important themes to glean from this definition. First, assessment is a process, rather than an outcome where students only have one attempt. Next, the primary function or purpose is on improving student learning; as such, assessment is a part of teaching and learning, not ancillary to it. Assessment also involves setting clear goals and determining effective methods to find out whether goals have been reached. Finally, teaching, learning and assessment are part of a bigger purpose and pattern on campus, and should not be done in isolation. Yet often assessment is talked about as if it is something we can decontextualize from universities, curriculum design, subject area, tutors and students. It is only in examining our assumptions, theories and practices that we can begin to understand how to gain some kind of alignment between learning and assessment.

Assumptions about assessment

Curricula where problem-based learning is central to the learning are largely constructivist in nature because students make decisions about what counts as knowledge and knowing. However, what continually undermines such learning are the assessment processes, which at worst are surveillance games and at best would appear to meet some of the ideals of constructive alignment that Biggs (1999) espouses (without necessarily being constructivist per se). Furthermore, assessment is rarely viewed as a process of development and for many students, failure is seen as devastation rather than a learning opportunity. Tutors tend to direct their students towards passing the module and encouraging them to be strategic rather than asking them to explore their own learning and position towards the knowledge on offer. Other difficulties with assessment in problem-based learning stem from tutors applying generalizable concepts and practices of assessment that fit with problem-based learning across diverse disciplines with different values and practices. In Appendix 1 we suggest several forms of assessment that we believe complement problem-based learning. Tutors need to find a fit between problem-based learning and the purpose and practice of assessment in the subject area in which it is being employed. Thus we argue for seven principles of assessment that support the underlying philosophies of this approach. These are as follows:

1   The assessment of student learning should begin with an exploration of educational values.
2   Assessment should reflect an understanding of learning as a multi-dimensional process.
3   It is important to ensure that there is alignment between our objectives

and the students' anticipated learning outcomes, the learning and teaching methods adopted, and the assessment of learning – strategies, methods and criteria.

4   Assessment should be a judgement based on performance grounded in criterion-referenced evidence.
5   Assessment is something which takes place in a context and the criteria should reflect that context.
6   Assessment should reflect what the professional does in their practice, which is largely process-based professional activity, underpinned by appropriate knowledge, skills and attitudes.
7   All assessment should reflect the learner's development from a novice to an expert practitioner and so should be developmental throughout the programme of studies.

(based on Astin *et al.* nd; Woods, 2000; Macdonald and Savin-Baden 2003)

Unpacking assessment concepts

Although in making distinctions between types of assessment there is a danger of setting up oppositions that may necessarily vilify one approach and extol others, there is value in identifying some differences in philosophies behind the increasingly separate lines of thought.

Traditional assessment

This often involves students selecting a response from a list of options; and is grounded in the belief that knowledge is universal and that students can take in knowledge as it is disseminated. It also identifies process and product as separate functions. It sees assessment as something that is objective and neutral. In this view, the tutor is an authority and expert, and students accomplish learning individually. It basically sums up students' level of knowledge and comprehension (Anderson 1998). Traditional assessment may involve measures such as multiple-choice examinations, true or false questionnaires, or fill in the blank quizzes.

Authentic or alternative assessment

This assessment movement began in the 1980s and involves students creating a response to a question or problem. It is rooted in the premise that knowledge has multiple meanings that cannot be objectively measured; rather, knowledge must be understood through the subjective impressions of those who possess it. Students do not take in knowledge as it is given out, but rather reconstruct information as they pass it through a variety of filters. Processes and products are linked together, and assessment thus becomes a subjective and value-laden activity. Control in the learning environment is shared between student and tutor, and learning occurs through collaboration. Authentic assessment aims to sum up students' capabilities for analysis, synthesis and evaluation (Anderson 1998). Authentic or alternative assessment may involve outside evaluation by experts, content analysis of projects, focus groups interviews, journal or activity logs, peer evaluations and personal reflections. Authentic assessment has been important in highlighting the importance of assessment as a process rather than just a means of grading students. The crucial underlying premise of authentic assessment is that it values the thinking behind the process of the work as much as the finished product. Thus authentic assessments are expected to incorporate a wide variety of techniques 'designed to correspond as closely as possible to "real world" student experiences' (Custer 1994: 66), and are seen to have meaning in themselves when the learning they measure has value beyond the learning environment and is meaningful to the learner. Thus students may be asked to evaluate case studies, write definitions and defend them orally, perform role plays or have oral readings recorded on tape. Much of what has been proposed in linking problem-based learning with the authentic assessment movement is little more than those arguments and ideas presented by Boud in the 1980s (Boud 1985, 1986).

There also seems to be an authentic problem-based learning movement emerging, which appears to be arguing that problem-based learning is only really authentic if it follows the original model espoused by Barrows (see, for example, Wee and Kek 2002). The real difficulty with the arguments offered by those in the authentic assessment movement is that they seem to want assessment to be authentic, but they are concerned that the assessment might be subjective, and so adopt tutor-centred rating scales. This concern would appear to be at odds with a form of assessment that is designed to be (subjectively) meaningful to the learner. However, the authentic movement has highlighted the importance of emphasizing both the process and product when assessing students, and in particular has encouraged tutors to develop forms of assessment that are clear, concise and communicated well to the students.

Purpose of assessment

We suggest that assessment is of two types, formative and summative, which have different but interrelated functions. Formative assessment is done primarily for the purpose of improvement and is prospective in that changes may be made that will help the object of the assessment. It involves providing the object of the assessment with feedback to help develop habits and improve performance and is generally diagnostic, goal-directed, formative (done for the purpose of providing feedback), and it is private, often anonymous. However, while not designed for grading, regular ongoing formative assessment can make grading easier because the tutor has observed the process, the tasks and the outcomes, and has informed the students on their progress, so surprises do not occur. Ongoing assessment can be beneficial in problem-based learning as it provides individuals and teams with interim feedback on their progress and assurance that their team is on target. Summative assessment involves gathering evidence, is retrospective in that it happens after the fact and is primarily done for documentation, accountability and evaluation.

It is important to ensure not only that assessment is aligned with the module objectives and the learning and teaching approach adopted, in this case problem-based learning, but also to ask why the assessment is being done. For example, it could be to

- support learning (formative assessment);
- improve learning (formative assessment);
- measure learning and provide certification (summative assessment);
- assure standards (summative assessment).

Assessing learners and learning

One of the most frequently cited concerns with problem-based learning is whether process will give over to product; thus knowledge is an area that is often assessed in a problem-based learning environment. Many educators wonder whether students will develop the same level of knowledge in the problem-based learning seminar compared with a more traditional one. This is with good reason. If problem-based learning does not deliver on developing student knowledge and the ability to critique, tutors will not adopt the approach. Many studies have been done in medical schools that compare traditional and problem-based learning modules producing mixed results; most studies show no difference in student learning (for example Coles 1985; Albanese and Mitchell 1993; Vernon and Blake 1993). Another object of assessment is skills. Among other things, tutors using problem-based learning often wish to measure problem-solving skills, team skills, self-directed learning skills and communication skills. These skills, aimed at helping students to become life-long learners, are very desirable attributes for all problem-based learning team members. Studies have argued that problem-based learning is successful in improving clinical and problem-solving skills (Albanese and Mitchell 1993; Vernon and Blake 1993; Silen 2001). Yet many tutors still assume that transferable skills are those that are seen to be transferable between contexts, for example, learned in the university and transferred to the world of work. However, there needs to be a distinction made between transferable skills and the ability to transfer skills. Bridges (1993) has argued that transferable skills are those that may be deployed in a variety of settings with little or no adaptation – such as word-processing skills.

Yet some skills are more context dependent (for example, the ability to negotiate) and require of the students more adaptation to the context than the simpler transferable skills such as word processing. Such adaptation demands meta-skills because students are required to adjust and apply their skills to different situations and social contexts. Many curricula today include transferable skills as part of the undergraduate programme, particularly in professional curricula. Courses in professional education have been the single highest growth area in UK higher education since the 1990s, due to the incorporation of professions such as nursing, occupational therapy and physiotherapy into the university system. This, along with the increasing links with industry, has meant that there has been an assumption that formal learning contexts can offer students opportunities to develop skills that are immediately transferable from the academic context to the work context. It could be said that students find the ability to do the transferring in the informal contexts as well, such as through debates in the coffee bars and practising presentation skills in their flats at the weekend.

A third object of assessment is *attitudes*. A general feeling pervades that education in general and problem-based learning specifically can and should be designed to change attitudes. Many tutors want to know if problem-based learning helps improve attitudes toward their subject matter, toward valuing opinions of others and toward willingness to engage in problem solving. However, the assessment of attitudinal change is notoriously difficult to achieve and the assessment of attitudes should focus on moving students towards a particular attitude rather than assigning a numerical value to attitudinal change. For example, students may be assessed on 'moving away from a view that there is a single body of correct knowledge, towards an understanding that knowledge is constructed and contestable', using criterion-referenced marking schemes.

When is assessment to occur?

Experience has often shown that if we adopt the 'big bang' approach to assessment at the end of a module, students will spend most of the team time with the facilitator trying to spot cues as to the assessment criteria and preferably, the answer that the facilitator wants! Yet more recent conceptions of assessment suggest that it should be ongoing and continuous.

Who is being assessed?

Proponents of the problem-based educational approach often believe that while good learning happens in problem-based teams, individual effort must be assessed, both to allow for individual accountability and to be able to assign a grade at the end of the module. In addition, there is an emerging group of tutors who use problem-based learning only with individual students and have no need to assess a non-existent team.

Who is going to carry out the assessment?

As we are giving greater responsibility to students for their own learning then it makes sense for them to take more responsibility for judging whether they have achieved the learning goals and have provided appropriate and adequate feedback. Similarly, given that they will be working with peers, supervisors and clients in professional capacities and assessment is matching the contexts in which professional capability will be demonstrated, the range of those involved in assessment and providing feedback needs to be extended. An often-asked question by a problem-based learning team is, 'Who will *do* the assessment?' Unlike on a traditional course where the lecturer is the only potential assessor, in a problem-based learning environment, where traditional lines of authority and control are turned on their heads, the list of potential assessors abounds. In addition, including assessors besides the facilitator furthers the goal of shared responsibility of learning, and makes it more likely that the facilitator may truly be seen as just that, if he or she has only partial or even no responsibility for assessment.

In addition to the facilitator, internal assessment can be carried out by students self-assessing themselves, or by student peers. Student peers will have worked closely together with the subject student in the problem-based environment and perhaps have the best ability to make an informed consideration about assessment. It has been shown that peer evaluations correlate highly with facilitator evaluation. In addition, a number of external assessors can provide useful assistance in the process. Having an external expert participate in assessment may add validity to the assessment experience, and having another tutor share assessment responsibilities can help to distribute the responsibility, making it less likely that the students will see the module facilitator as a punisher. An external team of peers may help make the experience more real for the students, and if the assessment is reciprocal, it may help students as they see the level of peers' work.

How is grading/marking to be done?

Grading represents a type of summative assessment. One of the tutor's decisions is whether to adopt norm-referenced or criterion-referenced grading. Norm-referenced grading (grading on the curve) can be particularly complicated in a collaborative team situation, because it involves comparing students to each other and thus fosters competition. If grades are norm-referenced, goals of positive interdependence and collaboration cannot be realized because students are placed in direct competition with each other; only a small percentage of the students can receive high grades. In other words, there are limited resources available. It is thus in the best interest of the individual student to hope that other students do poorly and remain confused. This grading scheme encourages the students to isolate themselves. On the other hand, using criterion-reference grading, in which the instructor sets defined criteria against which students will be evaluated, encourages collaboration by providing students with an incentive to help each other learn together. Many problem-based learning modules use pass/fail with a consequent greater emphasis on the feedback than summative accountability.

What feedback will students receive?

Will it be timely enough to help them learn and forward looking enough so as to help them move forward rather than just look back? Traditionally students have received little or no feedback on the major component of their assessment – examinations – adding to the pressure as it provides even less of a learning, and more of a measuring, purpose. Engaging with assessment criteria, and the use of self and peer assessment, will help improve the quality of feedback.

To date, research has been undertaken on assessment in the field of problem-based learning to ensure that the assessment of the students' performance in problem-based learning is consistent with the teaching method and to establish the effectiveness of problem-based learning. In particular these studies seek to establish that students are acquiring abilities in problem solving and professional competence.

Assessing teachers and teaching

The assessment of the problem-based learning facilitator is an interesting one. Evaluation of teaching has traditionally been done by way of a student rating or evaluation of the course and of the tutors. There are several common factors typically found in student rating forms (Centra 1993; Braskamp and Ory 1994): course organization and planning, clarity, communication skills, teacher–student interaction, rapport, course difficulty, workload, grading and examinations and student self-rated learning. Student ratings have proved good and valid measures of some aspects of teaching, in particular for tutor communication skills and for organization of material (Cashin 1990, 1995). However, traditional rating forms are just that: traditional. As such, they very often favour traditional teaching methods, because that is what they were designed to measure – whether the lecturer has done an effective job of presenting content and has tested the student on being able to memorize that content. Such evaluations do not necessarily carry out an effective job of assessing the myriad responsibilities of facilitators involved in designing an effective problem-based learning environment. These might include problem design to help students develop subject matter knowledge; curriculum development, which involves making sure that problems fit with other problems and courses fit with other courses; course design, so that the problem-based learning course helps students reach goals and objectives and so that accomplishment is effectively measured; providing appropriate resources so that students can solve the problem; being a resource and facilitator for student learning; carrying out administrative requirements, etc. These functions require a wide variety of context-specific measures to document effectiveness.

Evaluating facilitators

In terms of research into the evaluation of facilitators, Gijselaers and Schmidt (1990) found that tutor action had a direct causal influence on small group tutorials, which in turn influenced students' interest in the subject matter. These findings reflect the complexities involved in the facilitation of problem-based learning. Early studies by Dolmans *et al.* (1994a, 1994b) sought to quantify team facilitator behaviours and effectiveness, and a means of assessing tutor performance was developed in problem-based learning teams, but the scales made no allowance for the inclusion of personal attributes. Later Gijselaers (1997) examined contextual factors on tutors' behaviours and the effects of departmental affiliation on tutoring. Quantitative analysis of data indicated that overall the level of stability in tutor behaviour, which was examined across different problem-based learning teams, was low, as was the generalizability. What was apparent from the study, although Gijselaers did not couch it in such terms, was that both the learners and the learning context affected the team facilitator. Yet as Gijselaers (1997) discovered, much of what occurs in facilitating problem-based learning is related to the learners themselves. Such studies seem to imply a subtext about facilitation that has not been explored overtly in many of the quantitative studies. What we mean is that there appears to be an assumption that there are specific roles, attributes and ways of being that characterize facilitation that is 'good' or 'better' than others. Thus the idea that facilitation is a specific kind of 'role' is in itself problematic. It is as if there is some kind of idea of facilitators being able to construct a false identity in order to prevent themselves from becoming too subjective, too involved with students and their learning. Although it is perhaps inadvisable that the facilitator brings his own learning needs to the team discussion or attempts to create a culture of dependency in the team, to deny the inter-subjectivity of team and facilitator is somewhat naive.

We suggest that there are ways of helping tutors document as well as develop their facilitating expertise through a whole variety of evaluation processes that might include:

- *self-reflection*: such as self reports and course portfolios;
- *critique of materials*: such as syllabuses and course resource materials;
- *students*: such as student ratings of tutor development;
- *peers*: such as peer observation and interviews and peer interviewing of students;

- *instructional consultant*: such as videotaping the session and playing it back for a discussion.

Assessment and wider political concerns

If tutors get as far as being clear about the underlying purpose of assessment, they then have to examine the assumptions that go with particular disciplines. Those employed at a university are usually lecturers who teach within their discipline and utilize external examiners from that discipline. Thus the codes, practices and understandings of the discipline are maintained through teaching, assessment and quality mechanisms. Yet there is much to learn across different disciplines about the ways in which these disciplines use the same assessment. Furthermore, there are contradictions about many of the assumptions regarding assessment practices, such as the espousing of criterion-referenced assessment, and there are often detailed criteria to prove this. Yet when marking students' work, many tutors still subconsciously use norm-referenced approaches. While other tutors can argue against this and believe that they do not do it, the realities of this can been seen explicitly in the work of external examiners who acknowledge criterion-referenced marking, but still want to see a 'spread of marks across the year group'. Tutors' assumptions also become evident when they examine the types of answers that are deemed to be acceptable and those that are not. Many tutors feel uneasy about providing students with an assessment that encourages diverse answers and is difficult to mark. Even if tutors take such a risk, it is often difficult to uphold the marks they have given before their own peers, and subsequently to persuade their external examiners that such diversity is both fair and credible.

Heron (1989) has argued that the prevailing model for assessing students in higher education is thought to be an authoritarian one. Thus it is all a question of power, since traditional academic arguments suggest that students are not competent to participate in determining either their 'academic destiny' or their own competence. Such unilateral control by tutors is at odds with the process of education and ultimately breeds intellectual and vocational conformity in students. Heron has suggested that what is required is a redistribution of educational power, so that components of the curriculum become matters of tutor–student consultation. However, he expects that some components would be non-negotiable, as they represent educational principles that tutors believe are important and thus they are ones to which, as part of the module, students are invited to subscribe. Heron's arguments are persuasive and interesting, but in the current climate of performative values will be difficult to implement in some subjects. However, Usher and Edwards (1994) offer a further perspective on the issue of power in assessment of students' work. They have argued that some forms of continuous assessment, rather than being more student-centred than other traditional approaches to assessment, can be interpreted as a mechanism through which the process of surveillance is refined. What we see, in this situation, is that the students focus purely on the learning goals that are deeply embedded in the assessment criteria. Surveillance comes not necessarily through direct encounters with tutors, but through the performance criteria that appear to be empowering because they are available, and because students can see what they are expected to know. For example, it is expected that because students have the competences in their hands they will understand what to do and how to do it, and will thus be empowered. However, this too is problematic, since although they may look accessible, behavioural and achievable, 'competences are cast in behavioural terms but the discourse is itself not behaviourist. It is precisely because it is not, but rather interwoven with liberal humanist discourse that it is powerful' (Usher and Edwards 1994: 110). These kinds of codes and practices illustrate that in assessment the medium is also the message to the students, because it demonstrates to them what actually counts as knowledge and knowing in a given field. It seems puzzling that if tutors want to promote independence in inquiry and autonomy in learning, they so deeply mistrust students.

Conclusion

To conclude this section, we note that assessment in a problem-based learning environment can be challenging. It should focus on multiple skills and abilities, on process as well as product, and involve facilitators, students, external examiners and professional bodies. Many of the concerns about assessment in higher education seem to relate to the unintended side effects that undermine or contradict tutors' intentions to encourage students to learn effectively. It is essential, however, to develop a plan for assessment that fits within the module goals and the problem-based learning approach. Assessment in problem-based learning should be ongoing and over time, and should be contested ground where university and professional frameworks are interrupted by questioning academics who seek to enable students to learn through assessment as well as achieving a degree.

Part III

Broadening horizons

12

Embracing culture and diversity

Introduction

The issue of whether it is possible to use problem-based learning in all cultures and with a range of students is receiving increasing attention. There are ongoing discussions about whether cultural learning styles are a useful concept and reflections on the necessity of considering cultural issues when developing team ground rules. Many of these issues have been debated extensively, but to date little empirical evidence has supported or refuted the concerns raised. This chapter explores these issues and concerns and also examines some of the growing trends in the use of problem-based learning that raise questions about the cultural transferability of problem-based learning, namely exporting it from one culture to another. However we begin the chapter by examining the use of problem-based learning in non-dominant cultures.

Misplaced assumptions?

At both conferences and in journal articles in recent years there has been considerable discussion about whether it is possible or desirable to use problem-based learning in non-dominant cultures. The argument often heard is that problem-based learning does not work well with particular groups of students in specific countries. Yet when speaking with tutors from these countries who are using problem-based learning, many argue that it is the tutors who have difficulty in adapting and not the students. The focus to date has largely centred on Asian versus Western differences, yet there has been little research into other areas and this is reflected in the research and literature presented in this chapter. Furthermore, research by Eng (2000) and Khoo (2003) indicates that most students are able to adapt to problem-based learning. Eng (2000) suggests that since the Asian culture tends to emphasize loyalty and deference towards tutors, most students do not ask questions, are shy, lack self-esteem and fear being wrong. Thus, Eng argues, such 'Asian traits' appear to prevent the behaviour occurring that is necessary for implementing problem-based learning successfully; however, he suggests that environment can change this. Ahn (1999) surveyed Korean medical students on four-week postings to Canadian hospitals. After a week, the students became comfortable with learning through active and open dialogue, and the Canadian teachers found the Korean students were keen to learn through this approach. Eng (2000) confirmed these findings when problem-based learning was introduced at the National University of Singapore School of Medicine where, despite students' prior experience of a traditional school curriculum, they were able to adapt when placed in a different educational environment.

Khoo (2003) investigated the implementation of problem-based learning in Asian medical schools since he believed that there had been little research into whether the outcomes expected of the learner in problem-based learning were applicable to students from different cultural backgrounds. The result of examining conference presentations and published reports on this subject revealed that Asian medical students' experiences mirrored those of students in non-Asian medical schools. This study was particularly interesting in that it found, like so many other studies in the field of problem-based learning in general, that the design of the programme and the support and training for both tutors and students were the key factors in the successful implementation of problem-based learning. Furthermore, although MacKinnon (1999) argued that in Hong Kong the culture and local education system contributes to students' passive learning style, she also pointed out that:

> One of the most important lessons to be learned from the Hong Kong experience is that students seem to have less difficulty adapting to a PBL curriculum than do academic staff. We found that students' ability to transcend their cultural inhibitions and prior educational experiences was related to how well the conversion was managed. The challenge, therefore, lies in properly managing the process of curriculum reform.
>
> (MacKinnon 1999)

Similarly, work by Chung and Chow (2000) indicated that students found less difficulty adapting to problem-based learning than tutors and that both students' ability to transcend cultural inhibitions and their prior educational experiences related to how well the transition to problem-based learning was managed. Thus it would seem that concerns regarding the implementation of problem-based learning in particular cultures relate more to managing the process of curriculum reform than cultural adaptation per se.

Gender concerns

Although there have been many comparisons of the ways female and male students learn and function in education (for example, Gilligan 1979;

Belenky *et al.* 1986; hooks 1989; Orenstein 1994; Sadker and Sadker 1994), there have been relatively few studies into gender and problem-based learning. Most of the studies that have been undertaken have found little significant differences in male and female student responses to problem-based learning. For example, Cox (1996) studied 107 medical students in Trinidad and found that men tended to enjoy the problem-based learning sessions more than women and that racial or sexual discrimination by tutors towards students was reported by 29 per cent of the women in the study. Duek (2000) also studied medical students, but at the University of California at Los Angeles. She explored the quality of interactions in problem-based learning teams in a basic sciences module. The findings indicated that many female students relied on the tutor to ensure effective team management and: 'tutors' feedback, which can serve to reinforce or to redistribute status in the group ... appeared to be distributed in a manner that served to reinforce the status quo. If members of some ethnic groups are selectively not empowered in this manner, this may be one force acting to marginalize their participation ...' (Duek 2000: 104).

A recent study by Reynolds compared male and female views of participating in a problem-based module for occupational therapy and physiotherapy students at Brunel University, UK (Reynolds 2003). Although she found no significant differences attributable to gender with regard to students' experiences of problem-based learning, she did find small significant differences that indicated that women trusted information provided by other students more than men. They also showed that women enjoyed both the greater responsibility for their own learning and working with students from another therapy course, whereas the men showed more preference for lectures. However, Das Carlo *et al.* (2003) explored medical students' perceptions of what affected the productivity of problem-based learning teams and did note significant differences between male and female teams. However, they also pointed out the importance of taking account of cultural issues when setting the ground rules for tutorials. Some years ago Belenky *et al.* argued, 'Even when the context of the coursework includes issues of concern to women, strategies of teaching and methods of evaluation are rarely examined by faculty to see if they are compatible with women's preferred styles of learning. Usually faculty assume that pedagogical techniques appropriate for men are suitable for women' (Belenky *et al.* 1986: 5).

The difficulties with the studies that have been exploring gender issues in problem-based learning are perhaps related to the tendency to focus on male and female perceptions of self, as demonstrated through questionnaire ratings rather than issues of voice in the learning context. For example, what women and men espouse though a questionnaire response is often very different from behaviour seen in the actual environment. Studies that have explored women's voices (Gilligan 1979; Belenky *et al.* 1986) are methodologically different from recent studies into gender and problem-based learning such as those undertaken by Cox (1996) and Brown *et al.* (2003). We argue that interpretive studies such as these, that explore the ways in which women and men position themselves personally, pedagogically and interactionally in the learning environments, are vital in illuminating an in-depth understanding of gender differences in problem-based learning.

Using problem-based learning with 'less able' students

There have also been discussions about whether it is possible to use this approach with 'less able' students, who tend not to gain high grades in national school examinations, who lack confidence and who are considered by tutors to struggle in their courses either because of particular learning difficulties or because of poor study skills. Our experiences of curriculum reform both in the USA and the UK indicate that less able students value, enjoy and succeed in problem-based learning programmes because of the applied nature of the process. Furthermore, research into tutors' and students' experiences in two engineering programmes that adopted problem-based learning (Savin-Baden 2000) provides a comparative example:

> Gimmer[1] University was a traditional British university with a reputation for academic excellence. The problem-based learning course ran alongside conventionally taught modules in the third year of a BSc in mechanical engineering. Problem-based learning replaced a conventional lecture-based module on vibration that occurred in the third year of the traditional degree programme. The module was designed to promote a move away from the transmission of technical content and to enable students to develop skills in using new and previously learned material to engage with real engineering problem situations. Students on this programme tended to be white, middle-class British males, with top grades in science subjects from national schools examinations.
>
> Lembert University was a former polytechnic with a bias towards professional education. The BEng in Automotive Design (AMD) Engineering was a four-year sandwich course with the first year common with a BEng mechanical engineering degree. The approach in years 2 and 4 of the course was problem-based learning, the third year being the industrial placement. Students enrolled in the course having first selected whether to take the automotive engineering route or the conventional mechanical engineering degree. The specific automotive engineering aspects of the course were only introduced in the second year that centred around problem-based learning. Most of the students on this programme were males who had not obtained the grades to attend a higher-level university, or who had taken this degree because they were able to access the course with qualifications other than the standard qualifications (such as Higher National Diploma (HND), or equivalent qualifications), required by more traditional universities such as Gimmer.

Thus these two engineering programmes attracted students from markedly different social backgrounds, class and academic capability. Tutors in both institutions argued that problem-based learning suited their students, but for quite different reasons. At Gimmer problem-based learning helped promote a move away from the transmission of technical content and enabled students to develop problem-solving abilities and the application of content to problems in ways that were essential to engineering practice. In this module students were forced away from reproducing reports just based on a body of knowledge and instead were expected to develop professional skills, and the capacity to solve or manage real problems and present effective answers. At Lembert tutors argued that problem-based learning helped both able and less able students to develop confidence in their prior experience and use knowledge effectively, and found that students became increasingly self-directed as the course progressed. This, many tutors believed, was helped by self-assessment and peer assessment that were used to enable students to identify individual and group skills and attitudes.

The students themselves offered a variety of perspectives. Bill was a school leaver who had wanted to go to a university with more kudos than Lembert, but who did not achieve the grades required. Five ring binders full of information that he neither remembered nor understood symbolized his first year of dissonance on the mechanical engineering degree programme, which he was obliged to undertake before the more appealing applied AMD engineering course. Yet through the problem-based learning programme, an inner resonance with the material being learned emerged from his perception that it directly related to his future professional life. This stood in marked contrast to his feelings of estrangement from the first-year lecture material, which he felt to be irrelevant to his future career.

There were only two dissatisfied students; one at each university, who believed that problem-based learning did not suit the way in which they learned. Both of these students enjoyed and did well in examinations and both found collaborative learning difficult personally, but used particular mechanisms to ensure that they still did well in problem-based learning. Phil, a student at Gimmer, ensured that his marks were as high as possible by taking control of the team. It was he who collated and edited the team's written reports, and who took a lead in the team presentations. He had obtained high grades in his final school science exams and had been obliged to opt for the problem-based learning module in vibration engineering only because his final-year project was also in this subject. Throughout his degree he had chosen exam-based modules in order to 'get the best marks' and believed that any sense of enjoying and connecting personally with what was being learned was secondary to obtaining a good degree. Through knowledge of himself and his capacity as a 'skilled student', he distinguished studying from learning that might entail personal engagement, in order to read the system and make it work for him. Thus it would seem that students' prior experiences of learning and the particular view of learning they adopt largely affects their ability to engage with and manage problem-based learning.

Cultural learning styles and problem-based learning

Learning styles theory suggests that students prefer one way or style of learning over another, and thus if we design curricula in ways that fit with a variety of styles, then this may help to improve overall student achievement within a programme. The idea of cultural learning styles suggests that 'cultural upbringing plays a decisive role in determining a student's learning style' (Heredia 1999). However, before we engage with the notion of cultural learning styles, it is important to explore the relative value of learning styles per se. In recent years there has been critique of learning inventories that decontextualize learner and learning (for example Savin-Baden 2000; Haggis 2002), and that focus on particular characteristics of the learner rather than the person themselves. Haggis (2002) has suggested that over time the huge focus on the notion of deep and surface approaches to learning has resulted in assumptions being made that the study by Marton and Säljö (1984) had described a highly significant set of relationships about how students learn. This in turn has resulted in the promotion of types of learning environments that are expected to enhance deep approaches to learning – in many cases this would seem to be problem-based approaches. Although learners may change their approach according to their conception of the learning task, there is still an assumption that deep approaches are somehow necessarily better. As Haggis points out, many of these discussions about the promotion of 'deep approaches' seem to avoid the paradox that a surface approach can lead to successful learning and that changing one's approach is actually quite difficult. Many authors continue to suggest that problem-based learning promotes deep approaches (as opposed to surface or strategic approaches) to learning, the underlying assumption being that this is necessarily a good thing. There does appear to be some conflict around the notion of developing a deep approach, in that approaches are difficult to change and in many instances surface approaches can result in very successful learning.

In recent years studies have attempted to identify learning style preferences among students from a variety of cultures. Table 12.1 is adapted from the information provided by Heredia (1999) and MacKinnon (1999), and the recommendations suggest ways of engaging students in diversifying their learning. Interestingly, one of the recommendations made by those who have studied cultural learning styles is the use of cooperative learning for students from diverse cultural backgrounds. However, like the many learning styles inventories, the idea of cultural learning styles seems to rather oversimplify the issues, and the studies in this field indicate this through the contradictory research findings available (for example, Guild and Garger 1998; Hilliard 1988; Irvine and York 1995).

Table 12.1 Cultural learning styles

Type of student	Preference	Recommendation to diversify learning
Hispanic	Conformity, peer-orientated learning, kinaesthetic instruction resources, high degree of structure, a field-dependent cognitive style	Cooperative learning, use of humour, drama, modelling and a global rather than an analytic approach to understanding
African American	Inferential reasoning, focus on people rather than things, kinaesthetic learning, more proficient in non-verbal communication	Loosely structured learning environment with tutor working with students
Native American	Field-dependent, visual rather than verbal information, learning in private rather than public, learning by watching and doing, value in concise speech	Minimized lecturing and teacher direction, reduced competition and focus less on individual achievement
Asian	High educational attainment, conformity, high degree of structure, low participation in class, modelling, to be supplied with large amount of written information	Cooperative learning, a global rather than an analytic approach to understanding, encourage questioning
Western European	Preference for working alone, values guided learning but also structured debate. Tendency to focus on linguistic capability and individual attainment.	Loose structure to learning context, promote cooperative learning and minimize lecturing and dependence on tutor

Considering cultural issues when implementing problem-based learning

Our experience of working with tutors in different universities suggests that the consideration of cultural issues when forming problem-based learning teams and asking them to develop team ground rules is an area that is often overlooked by both tutors and students. A colleague was facilitating problem-based learning in a Scottish university where all but one of the students in the team was Scottish. This lone Irish student had considerable difficulty in understanding the team discussion because of the other students' accents. The Irish student's inability to understand was misconstrued by the other members as non-commitment to the team until the student pointed out the problem. This shocked the Scottish students and prompted them to consider the way in which their assumptions about their own culture and values might affect their roles as future professionals. This example had a positive ending but this may not always be the case. Yet it is important to consider the team mix when deciding on problem-based learning teams, something we dealt with earlier in Chapter 7. There are, however, few studies in this area and it seems even fewer into the relative relevance of cultural learning styles and problem-based learning.

Using problem-based learning to teach students about cultural issues

Many programmes that have adopted problem-based learning include within the problem scenario issues that raise cultural awareness in students. Some programmes, however, put particular emphasis on cultural concerns and have specific problems to address these concerns. For example, students are enabled to learn about cultural minority groups by collecting data about a particular group and then verifying it with that group or individual representing that group (see, for example, Ojanlatva *et al.* 1997).

Crossing cultural boundaries with problem-based learning programmes

Online learning and distance education have been huge areas of development since the late 1980s. Although distance education is often used to support learners who cannot always attend the university for face-to-face contact or those who live far from the university, there has been a shift in recent years toward exporting programmes from one country to another. In such cases distance learning becomes a more complex activity than the idea that learning just takes place removed from the tutor in both time and space, since cultural differences come to the fore in these new exported programmes.

Currently, there are modules and programmes that use different forms of online learning to support problem-based learning but few, if any, to date that are wholly problem-based. Using computer-mediated communication with distance learners was initially seen as having the ideal of 'a collaborative respectful interdependence where the student takes responsibility for personal meaning as well as creating mutual understanding in a learning community' (Garrison 1993: 17). Given that in problem-based learning collaborative learning is seen as one of the key features of the approach, it might seem at first that computer-mediated problem-based learning is a retrograde step. There is a certain sense that working and learning face-to-face in teams is vital to the whole process of problem-based learning. Using problem-based learning at a distant computer can help students to use team conferences as a central communication space, and as a place both for sharing and examining individual perspectives and managing the work and administration of the team interaction.

There are currently a number of different ways in which problem-based learning is being used at a distance and these can be defined as follows:

- computer-mediated collaborative problem-based learning;
- migrated programmes;
- exported problem-based learning;
- transnational problem-based learning.

Computer-mediated collaborative problem-based learning

Computer-mediated collaborative problem-based learning is defined here as students working in teams of 8–10 on a series of problem scenarios that combine to make up a module. Students are expected to work collaboratively to solve or manage the problem. Students will work in real-time or asynchronously, but what is important is that they work together. Synchronous collaboration tools are vital for the effective use of computer-mediated collaborative problem-based learning, and tools such as Chat, Shared Whiteboards, Video conferencing and Group browsing are central to ensuring collaboration within the problem-based learning team.

Students may be working at a distance or on campus, but they will begin by working out what they need to learn to engage with the problem situation. This may take place through a shared whiteboard, conferring or an e-mail discussion group. What is also important is that students have both access to the objectives of the module and also the ability to negotiate their own learning needs in the context of the given outcomes. Facilitation occurs through the tutor having access to the ongoing discussions without necessarily participating in them. Tutors also plan real-time sessions with the computer-mediated collaborative problem-based learning team in order to engage with the discussion and facilitate the learning. An example of such a form of computer-mediated collaborative problem-based learning can be seen at Glasgow Caledonian University. This is a one-year conversion course for qualified nurses who require the further qualification of mental health nurse, and is undertaken at a distance.

Migrated problem-based learning

Here programmes are transferred from one university to another in the same country. What usually occurs is that one university develops a problem-based learning programme within a given discipline, and then packages it so that is can be sold to another. Some such programmes have been successful in the UK, but many tutors have spent considerable time adapting the new programme to the local context and this has been a demanding and time consuming approach. What is becoming more common is the purchasing or exchanging of problem scenarios between disciplines often facilitated by either an external consultant or a website.

Exported problem-based learning

To date there have been several problem-based learning programmes that have been exported and then subsequently adapted by the buying country's tutors. The University of Sydney and Flinders University, Australia, have both successfully exported their medical programmes to UK universities. The difficulty here for many universities is the cost of buying such programmes. Few can afford to purchase them even though they are well designed and well thought through programmes. The other difficulty is that even when transferred across Western cultures they still need further adaptation to fit the local context, and this inevitably requires further funding. However, the programmes from Sydney and Flinders were adapted for graduate-entry medical programmes that needed to be developed quickly, and the adaptation to date appears to have been very successful.

Transnational problem-based learning

Transnational problem-based learning refers to the delivery of a programme at a distance to students in a country other then the offering institution, where the offering institution largely supports and adapts the programme. Such programmes are increasingly common in the distance education arena but are still relatively recent in the global problem-based learning community. Conway *et al.* (2000) document their experience of delivering an Australian nursing curriculum in the Maldives. The issues they suggest that need careful consideration are the difference in beliefs and attitudes about illness and healthcare, and the differences and values placed on cultural religious traditions.

This paper raised the interesting question of the extent to which the processes embedded in problem-based learning were universally relevant. It is clearly a question that requires further exploration but certainly many of those working with Asian students have argued that such processes are relevant to them. However, we would suggest that transnational problem-based learning should be tailored to the specific cultural context of the students even though some tutors may suggest, with Biggs (1997), that cultural difference can be overcome by applying universal principles of good teaching, regardless of where the programme is taught.

Equipping staff for facilitation in diverse contexts

In some universities, something that we would refer to as small group teaching is referred to as problem-based learning. Additionally, students working in groups of four in a tiered lectured theatre, discussing questions the lecturer has raised following a short talk he has given, has also been termed problem-based learning, whereas we would see this as an interactive lecture. The lines between different forms of interactive learning, small group teaching and problem-based learning will inevitably remain blurred. However, it is important to understand the purpose for which we are equipping facilitators. Although it is important for all facilitators to undergo educational development at the outset, dealing with different constructions of problem-based learning demands different capabilities. For example, if students in a first-year module are undertaking problem-based learning with a large cohort of students (150–80), and it has been decided to conduct it in a large room with students in teams of five around tables with a roving facilitator, then this facilitator will need to be equipped for such an approach. One facilitator managing a single team of 10 students in one dedicated room is a completely different challenge. Small team problem-based learning can result in an intense and sometimes co-dependent relationship between facilitator and team; confusion can arise between the role of the facilitator and that of the personal tutor, so that lines become blurred between students' personal and pedagogical problems.

In contrast, in large-team, problem-based learning there are opportunities for students to avoid undertaking the work, individually or corporately, attendance is difficult to monitor, the room will be noisy and the facilitator will be required to facilitate many small teams all at the same time, with feedback becoming complex and difficult. It is therefore important when designing any module that the educational development provided prepares facilitators for either a range of ways of utilizing problem-based learning or is specifically focused on the type to be used.

However, there would appear to be a number of issues that need to be considered when working with students who are from cultures where the tutor–student relationships are traditionally hierarchical, where tutors are revered for their knowledge and where students' educational attainment will necessarily affect their family's social mobility and economic security. In such cases it is important to recognize that students will need to be encouraged to challenge tutors, but that this should be done in stages so that trust is built up between tutors and students. It is also important to help students to understand the value of deep approaches to learning so that they see that such approaches aid long-term memorization. In many Asian cultures surface approaches to learning tend to be reinforced by competitive education systems that have large classes, didactic lectures and plenty of handouts. Making mistakes, getting it wrong and reluctance to speak for fear of being seen as arrogant are all difficult issues to deal with in helping students to move towards problem-based learning. However, discussing students' concerns with them and perhaps using a problem-solving approach first can help them to adapt to becoming independent inquirers who own their own learning experiences.

Conclusion

Dealing with cultural concerns in problem-based learning is no different from dealing with them in other areas of the curriculum: it requires sound preparation, awareness of students with difficulties, sensitivity to differences and honesty with ourselves and our students about what is possible within the organization and culture where we are operating. Research is still required concerning the use and success of transnational problem-based learning and regarding whether particular models of problem-based learning or modes of curriculum practice tend to fit better into some cultural contexts than others.

Note

1   The names of the universities here are pseudonyms.

13

Programme evaluation

Introduction

Many aspects of problem-based learning programmes may be evaluated using a variety of methods. In this chapter, we consider the concept of programme evaluation and begin by establishing some basic definitions and reviewing some common models. We continue the chapter moving into an analysis of the methods and instruments often used to evaluate problem-based learning programmes, and then we present some findings from recent evaluation studies. The section ends as we consider some common concerns when evaluating problem-based learning programmes and address some of the myths about programme evaluation.

Purposes and goals of evaluating problem-based learning programmes

To evaluate something is to determine or fix the value of it. While many see evaluation as determining significance, worth, or condition of changes in behaviour, performance and competencies, we rather hold the view that you should *assess people* and *evaluate things*. In the case of problem-based learning, we believe we should assess students and facilitators, but we should evaluate problem-based learning programmes. Therefore, we define evaluation as something done to determine the effectiveness of programmes and projects designed to produce change that is carried out by careful appraisal and study. Cox *et al.* (1981) suggest a number of styles and dimension of evaluation, which we include in Figure 13.1.

Evaluation of a problem-based learning programme involves collecting information which can include programme goals and the structure of the curriculum, connections with student needs, scholarly inquiry or other disciplines; teaching quality, advising, inclusiveness, institutional support and

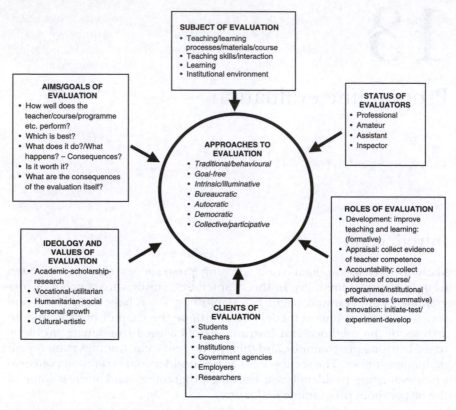

Figure 13.1   Styles and dimensions of evaluation
(Adapted from Cox *et al.* 1981)

outcomes. Such evaluation tends to examine the conceptualization, design, implementation and usefulness of the programme. It can be undertaken in order to make effective decisions about a programme – formative evaluation. As the approach grows and develops, information that can be used for improvement purposes can provide valuable directions and ways forward for the approach. Evaluation may lead stakeholders to understand the influence of the approach on learning outcomes and on student experiences. It can aid problem-based learning to be more efficient in different contexts and hopefully also make it less costly. It can help institutions and tutors determine whether the approach is really doing what they planned. Evaluation can improve administration's understanding of the wider programme's goals and how problem-based learning is helping to meet those goals. It can be used in a programme's documentation to increase its validity for export elsewhere.

Problem-based learning programmes are also evaluated to provide accountability – summative evaluation, to show that such programmes are *at least* as effective as more traditional programmes. For example, information for accountability purposes is helpful in showing that problem-based learning is an effective educational approach and can be used to improve public relations. From our perspective, though, summative evaluations have limited usefulness for problem-based learning. While this kind of evaluation is usually carried out to aid improvement in traditional programmes, it is not really possible to do the same in problem-based learning programmes, as they are not pursuing similar objectives.

Models of evaluation

There are a myriad of evaluation models, and while a review of all models is beyond the scope of this chapter, we believe it useful to identify some of the models that have been used to evaluate problem-based learning programmes so far, as well as some that have potential for use in the future. Evaluation models all have distinct purposes and uses, some of which are more appropriate for problem-based learning than others.

The *traditional evaluation* model was perhaps born out of the work of the educational psychologist Tyler (1969). Such evaluation involves stating goals and objectives in behavioural terms, developing measurement instruments, measuring achievement of goals and objectives, comparing objectives and achievement, interpreting findings and making recommendations (Stark and Lattuca 1997). This model may be criticized for its overt emphasis on behavioural objectives and mechanistic procedures for evaluation, and as such has particularly limited usefulness for problem-based learning, but it did provide educators with one of the first systematic models for measuring programme effectiveness.

The *professional expert* model (Stark and Lattuca 1997: 285) falls within the accreditation tradition. In this model, the expert proposes standards, obtains agreement from other relevant peer experts, requires self-study against standards, has peer experts examine the self-study, reports on the examination and has peer experts determine whether standards have been met. This model also has limited usefulness for problem-based learning because it fails to involve stakeholders and it relies on standards set by an external agent. However, given the increased calls for accountability, it is a reality in higher education and thus cannot be ignored.

The *countenance model*, perhaps best described by Stake (1978), is descriptive in nature and looks at prior conditions or antecedents, implementation or transactions, and outcomes. It is in keeping with Astin's I-E-O model (inputs, environment, outcomes). It has some usefulness in problem-based learning when evaluators want to know what outcomes are related directly to the experience.

The *Context, Inputs, Process, Products (CIPP)* model, as described by Stufflebeam (2000), is again descriptive and focuses on describing programme goals, design, implementation and outcomes. This model has more relevance to problem-based learning as it focuses on process and acknowledges context.

Goal-free evaluation describes programmes and improvement and Scriven (1972) suggests that it occurs when the evaluators are not cued to the programme's goals. Scriven's model has some interesting implications for problem-based learning programmes that tend to have overt goals that drive the programme development. Few studies have used this model, but it would be interesting to see the results of an evaluation in which the evaluators were not cued into the goals of the programme. How would problem-based learning fare?

Experimental evaluation is carried out for basic research and accountability. This type of evaluation intends to add back to the knowledge base. While research for research's sake is important to a degree, it is also desirable to add back to the knowledge base, and this type of evaluation of problem-based learning programmes should then add value to them.

Illuminative evaluation increases understanding and describes programmes. It focuses on the actual learning situation, or the learning milieu (Parlett and Deardon 1977) and is conducted in three overlapping stages of observing, inquiring and then seeking explanations. This method can increase our knowledge of the issues connected with the types of problems used, context in which problem-based learning has been implemented and facilitator–student dynamics.

A final model is *naturalistic evaluation*, described by Lincoln and Guba (1985). This model involves gathering descriptive information regarding the evaluation object, setting, surrounding conditions, relevant issues, and values and standards for worth and merit; determining information desired by and sharing with relevant audiences; and negotiating decisions. This model, with its focus on collaboration and negotiation, is perhaps the most useful for problem-based learning because it involves collaboration with participants and is based upon their lived experiences.

To summarize, traditional models of evaluation, which tend to be strictly quantitative and summative in nature, have limited usefulness for problem-based learning. We believe that some of the more naturalistic methods which contain more qualitative, interpretative and collaborative inquiry and which are done to illuminate, to improve understanding and awareness and to respond to varied needs hold more promise for problem-based learning.

Methods for evaluating problem-based learning programmes

Many methods have been used to evaluate problem-based learning programmes, and the following represent the methods we suggest:

Questionnaires, surveys, checklists

These methods are often used when information is needed quickly. They are a useful way to get information from a large number of people in a non-threatening way. They have the advantage of being anonymous, inexpensive and easy to analyse. In addition many previously validated instruments exist. Examples of this include the Course Experience Questionnaire (CEQ) developed by Ramsden and colleagues (Ramsden 1991), designed to measure the quality of the student learning experience, and the Student Course Experience Questionnaire (SCEQ). These methods may not provide deep or careful feedback, as the wording of the instruments can bias the responder's comments, they can be very impersonal and restricting, and, thus, not always provide the full story. Despite the pitfalls, to date, these have been the most common methods of evaluation used in problem-based learning programmes.

Interviews

Interviews are used when researchers want to fully understand impressions or experiences. This method can often provide rich and satisfying information to help unpack the problem-based learning experience from the perspective of the participants. They may also be collaborative methods of inquiry, which lend authenticity. However, this method takes time and so can be costly. It can also be difficult to analyse and compare.

Document reviews

This method is used when an impression of how the programme operates is desired. It can take the form of an unobtrusive review of documents such as memos, minutes from meetings and syllabuses. It has the advantage of not interrupting the programme and not biasing respondents. It can provide comprehensive and historical information and is inexpensive, as the data already exists. However, it can take time and may provide an incomplete picture, as data are restricted to existing forms.

Observations

Observations have been used to gather information about how a programme operates, and particularly focuses on process. It has the advantage of evaluating the programme as it is unfolding and it can be adapted as events occur. It can be filed to preserve a permanent record of the process and it can be played back to individuals for review and comment. However, it is often difficult to interpret and categorize observed behaviours, and the very fact of being observed can influence individual behaviours.

Focus groups

Focus groups provide in-depth information about a programme. They are a good way to get common impressions and can elicit significant information in a short time. They also have a social aspect that may elicit more responses than a one-to-one interview might. However, peer pressure can change perspectives, and it can be hard to analyse data.

Nominal Group Technique

Nominal Group Technique is helpful in identifying problems, exploring solutions and establishing priorities. It typically includes four steps:

1   Silent generation of ideas in writing: Participants independently write down their responses to a stimulus question.
2   Round-robin recording of ideas: Each participant contributes a single idea that is recorded on a board; discussion of the ideas is not permitted; and the process continues until there are no more ideas.
3   Discussion of the list of ideas: Participants discuss each idea in turn so that they are clear about its meaning.
4   Voting: Participants individually rank the five ideas they like best, scoring them from 1 to 5; votes are recorded on the board and the idea with the best total is selected.

The final product consists of a decision and a list of the ideas that were generated. Because the technique includes a voting procedure, the group members feel they have arrived at their decision through consensus. However, it is difficult to craft the appropriate stimulus question. This technique is also not suitable for all questions, and is time intensive (Brassard 1989: 91–3).

Case studies

Case studies are perhaps the most comprehensive way to evaluate a programme. They involve multiple data points, which may include participant interviews, focus groups, document analysis, field notes and direct observation. Case studies may also directly involve participants so that inquiry becomes more collaborative in nature. They may be exploratory, explanatory or descriptive. Whatever the purpose, case studies provide in-depth, detailed, rich and descriptive information about a programme. Recent innovations in research methodology have added rigour to case-study methodology, by setting new standards for data trustworthiness and by setting a trend for undertaking multiple case studies that makes results more generalizable beyond the bounds of a single case. While case studies are time consuming to carry out, they are also a good way to portray a programme to outsiders.

Findings from evaluation studies in problem-based learning

Expected learning outcomes

Most of the current studies of problem-based learning programmes involve comparisons between problem-based and traditional approaches, seeking to evaluate outcomes. The first outcome usually explored is *knowledge*. Many tutors have attempted to determine the effectiveness of problem-based learning programmes since the approach's inception in the 1960s, with much of the research conducted in medical schools. Student knowledge is one outcome that is frequently assessed. The results in this area have been mixed, with some studies showing slight increases in basic knowledge, some showing slight decreases, and the majority showing no significant differences (Albanese and Mitchell 1993; Vernon and Blake 1993). On some tests of medical knowledge, students in traditional programmes have scored higher than students in problem-based ones (Schmidt *et al.* 1987; de Vries *et al.* 1989), but as we see next, this is often offset by skills gained.

Additional studies have compared the effectiveness of problem-based and traditional curricula on developing lifelong learning skills. Several of these studies have specifically looked at clinical performance as a demonstration of these skills, and in most cases, problem-based learning students performed better than traditional learning students (Albanese and Mitchell 1993; Vernon and Blake 1993). Students who acquired knowledge in the context of solving problems were more likely to use it spontaneously to solve new problems than individuals who acquired the same information under the more traditional methods of learning facts and concepts through lectures (Bransford *et al.* 1989). In addition, it has been suggested that students in problem-based learning environments developed stronger clinical competencies although the differences were small and non-significant (de Vries *et al.* 1989). Furthermore, Moore *et al.* (1994) reported a statistically significant difference on an ethics problem-solving task undertaken with Harvard medical students. Another study conducted on a nutrition and dietetics course found that problem-based learning students perceived they developed stronger thinking and problem-solving skills than traditional learning students (Lieux 1996).

A second outcome usually considered is *learning process*. Several studies have found that students on problem-based learning courses have different approaches to research and reference processes. Often this difference is evident in the way that students obtain and use the tools of the discipline. Studies showed that problem-based learning medical students were most likely to use journals, online resources and to rely on informal discussion with their peers. They also used textbooks and other resources more than their traditional learning counterparts. Traditional learning students were most likely to rely on lecture notes. Medical problem-based learning students were also more likely to use the library, study within the library and make greater use of self-selected resources. In contrast, traditional learning medical students made more use of tutor-selected resources (for example, Blumberg and Michael 1992; Rankin 1992).

Several studies also demonstrate that problem-based learning affects students' approaches to learning; in particular, students on problem-based courses were more likely to use deep and strategic approaches than their traditional counterparts. Bernstein *et al.* (1995) noted that students reported problem-based learning facilitated thinking about material rather than simply memorizing it, showing that problem-based learning prompts deep approaches to learning. Similarly, Coles (1985) and Newble and Clarke (1986) used the Approaches to Studying Inventory developed by Entwistle *et al.* (1979) to verify that problem-based learning students were more likely to use versatile approaches to study for the meaning and less likely to use reproduction, again signifying more deep approaches. Nolte *et al.* (1988) found that use of reserve material went up, showing more strategic approaches to learning and Woodward and Ferrier (1982) found that McMaster graduates felt more competent in areas such as independent study, gathering data and problem-solving, but badly prepared in the basic medical sciences.

Problem-based learning has been shown to develop a host of other outcomes. For example, student retention among medical school students in The Netherlands improved, with students in the problem-based learning medical programme being much more likely to graduate and to do so in less time than students in the more traditional curriculum (de Vries *et al.* 1989).

Problem-based learning would also appear to enhance team skills. Cockrell *et al.* (2000) conducted a study on college graduates, in which they examined students' perspectives on their learning as members of collaborative teams. The researchers found that students used negotiation to mediate differences and maintain a healthy collaborative environment. The researchers suggested that within the teams, leadership moved from student to student as situations arose and were resolved. Team members also held each other accountable for achieving learning goals. Finally, team members validated team and individual learning. They also found that problem-based learning fostered students' sense of ownership of the knowledge that was created over the course. Problem-based learning students also developed more of a sense of personal responsibility than did students who received lectures (Lieux 1996). In addition, Andersen and McMillan (1991) carried out a longitudinal study of graduates, finding that they were autonomous in their practice, responsible and accountable, self-reflective and assertive, showed evidence of ongoing learning, were less self-conscious than hospital-based peers, and used a problem-solving strategy to identify people's needs.

Student experiences

Evidence suggests that students' attitudes toward learning improve in a problem-based learning programme. In a study conducted at the University of Toronto Faculty of Medicine, for example, researchers evaluated shifts in students' attitudes after initial direct experience with problem-based learning (Bernstein *et al.* 1995). Questionnaires were administered at the beginning of the first problem-based learning session and at the close of the last session (five weeks later) to the 250 second-year students. Between the pre-test and post-test there was a statistically significant increase from 38 per cent to 52 per cent in the students' perceptions that, overall, problem-based learning methods were more effective than traditional teaching methods. While the students rated traditional methods as better for knowledge acquisition, they rated problem-based learning methods better for improving teamwork and doctor–patient relationships. Students perceived the advantages of problem-based learning to be that it was more stimulating and enjoyable, and that it taught them how to learn rather than how to memorize. At post-test, there was an increase in favourable comments by the students. Thus, direct experience with problem-based learning led to more favourable attitudes among the students.

Students also often report greater satisfaction with their experiences. For example, problem-based learning medical students at Harvard reported that their studies were more engaging, difficult and useful than non-problem-based learning students (Albanese and Mitchell 1993). Vernon and Blake (1993) carried out a review of all the available evaluative research from 1970 to 1992 that compared problem-based learning programmes with more traditional ones. They found that students' attitudes and opinions about problem-based learning were more positive than those on traditional programmes. In addition, Schmidt *et al.* (1987) reviewed 15 studies that compared various educational outcomes of problem-based learning. They concluded that problem-based learning curricula provided a student-centred learning environment and encouraged curiosity in learning, whereas more traditional programmes produced students who used rote memorization and short-term learning strategies.

Tutor knowledge and experiences

Surprisingly few studies have focused on tutors' outcomes or experiences with problem-based learning. Studies conducted by Major and Palmer (2002) showed that tutors who move from traditional teaching to a problem-based learning environment do change their knowledge levels in several important ways. They change their views of themselves as teachers, shifting away from an authoritarian perspective. In addition, facilitators change their views of their students, coming to accept them as peers and professionals. Facilitators change their knowledge of their fields, starting to see inter and intra disciplinary connections they had been unaware of previously. Finally, they change their knowledge of instructional methods and strategies, expressing the value of educational techniques such as scaffolding. Scaffolding involves coaching students to become independent inquirers, by designing problems and activities to enable them to overcome gaps in their knowledge and capabilities. Turpie and Blumberg (1999) found that problem-based learning tutors believed that they had learned more about their subject from students' discussions, particularly in areas outside their fields of expertise. They also developed new ways to learn subject matter from these experiences, such as conducting literature searches and using the internet. Some evidence does show that many tutors' experiences with problem-based learning are positive. Tutors who are familiar with problem-based learning favour it over other methods. For example, Dahlgren *et al.* (1998) found that tutors' perceptions of their roles influenced their levels of satisfaction. Tutors who perceived themselves as supporters, emphasized the responsibilities of the students and those who spent more time on group process were more satisfied with the problem-based learning experience than their non-supportive peers, who instead viewed themselves as directors.

Continuing questions about evaluation studies

While many studies point to improved outcomes and experiences, questions about the evaluations are still of concern. For example, Norman and Schmidt (1992) point to empirical evidence supporting the fact that when prior knowledge is activated, learning is improved, and when knowledge is elaborated, later retrieval is improved. Evenson and Hmelo (2000) however, argue that their theory is vague and lacks empirical evidence. Berkson (1993), Woodward (1997) and Colliver (2000) argue that many studies erroneously claim effects for problem-based learning when it is more likely that the effects were due to differences in sample selection and philosophy of care. Davies (2000) argues that it seems safe to conclude that problem-based learning may not be invariably better than other methods, or superior for all types of learning or learners. We suggest that we need stronger evidence that problem-based learning improves learning and experiences and that the studies must be well designed and valuable.

Issues in programme evaluation

Many early evaluation studies focused on comparing the outcomes of problem-based learning approaches against those of more traditional pedagogical methods. There are some signs of positive change, and these often occur because of the inclusion of more qualitative and collaborative inquiry. However there remain a number of obstacles to be overcome:

- *Effects of the process.* Evaluation is intrusive and can change participant's perspectives. This is sometimes referred to as the Hawthorne effect, in which observation and study initially create improved processes and products, as participants are singled out and made to feel important. Yet many who have undertaken longitudinal studies would argue either that this is not the case or that it is an arrogant presumption to believe that the researcher can really have that much impact on participant behaviour.

- *Socio-political issues.* We argue that all evaluation at its heart has a socio-political aspect. The evaluation is done to increase awareness, but on many occasions stakeholders are wary of receiving a complete evaluation that may have partially undesirable results that will interfere with public relations and funding. It is important to make decisions about the scope of the evaluation and dissemination plans in advance.

- *Ethics.* One of the difficulties in evaluation is the way that the information discovered is then actually used by evaluators, participants and university administrators. If the evaluators are to be considered trustworthy they must protect those being evaluated from harm. The consequence may mean that some information is not used. This is rather reminiscent of the question, 'Whose side are we on?' (Becker 1970: 99), and the evaluation debates relating to who is saying what about whom. Ethics must always be considered in evaluation and the principles of autonomy, informed consent, non-maleficence and beneficence should always be observed.

- *Trustworthiness.* Trustworthiness is always an issue in any kind of qualitative evaluation. In quantitative studies, validity and reliability are at issue. Practices associated with trustworthiness and authenticity often include triangulation, member checking and reflexivity, that are all designed to ensure transparency and credibility in evaluation. However, we believe that what is required is a shift away from validity, trustworthiness and the assumption that we really can find shared truths. Instead we argue for 'honesties' (following Stronach *et al.* 2002) – a category that allows us to acknowledge that trust and truths are fragile, while at the same time enabling us to engage with the messiness and complexity of evaluation in ways that really do reflect the lives of our participants. Honesties is a more moral category because of the way it enables us to engage with the fragility and the instability of people and their contexts.

- *Who should carry out the evaluation?* The question of who should carry out the evaluation is an issue. An external expert can add credibility by providing an 'outsider' and 'objective' perspective. An insider such as a peer may know the situation better and thus may better be able to understand nuances of the data. Collaborative approaches may yield the best data but may be questioned by those with strongly embedded quantitative perspectives.

- *Mirroring practice.* One common concern about evaluation of problem-based learning programmes is that it so rarely matches practice. As we argued in Chapter 3, problem-based learning represents a constructivist approach, and traditional evaluation methods may not enable us to capture the many facets of this educational approach. This is changing to some extent with the use of more naturalistic and collaborative modes of inquiry.

Myths about programme evaluation for problem-based learning

Many myths about programme evaluation exist (Patton 1991), and many of these are applicable to problem-based learning.

Evaluation should involve quantitative design and data

Traditional programme evaluation emerged as a quantitative model, and that model has stuck over time. These evaluations give the perception of scientific accuracy, but are as biased as qualitative examinations, since evaluators still determine what questions are included, how they are worded and so forth. Newer methods of inquiry are providing richness and depth to our understanding of problem-based learning. In addition, we are beginning to understand programme evaluation as a process and not as merely findings.

Outcomes are too difficult to measure

Part of the concern with problem-based learning programme evaluation has been that outcomes are fuzzy and, therefore, difficult to measure. This myth stems from older notions about evaluation that rely on experimental design and comparisons between problem-based learning and traditional learning programmes. However, many indirect and 'softer' measures can provide good and useful information about outcomes in easy to access and inexpensive ways.

Evaluation should prove success or failure of a programme

Many people believe that evaluation is about proving the success or failure of a programme. However, this assumes a perfect programme, which is not a reality. More recently, evaluation has begun to be seen not only as a one-shot approach or episodic but rather as something that is continuous and ongoing. Furthermore, perspectives about the nature of evidence are on the move, as Barnett notes:

A changing world is one of non-replicability. Tomorrow will not be like today . . . if we are not careful, basing practice on evidence may serve the purpose of locking us into undesirable practices that should have been jettisoned with the ark . . . more than 'evidence' is required. Also required are imaginative ideas and value judgments as to what is to count as desirable. It may be, then, that the real value of evidence in relation to practice is to guide us away from certain kinds of practice rather than towards certain kinds of practice.

(Barnett 2001)

Generalizations and recommendations should be avoided

For many years, evaluation was viewed as something that should be neutral and objective. However, recent trends in learning theory have led us to hold more proactive stances in both our methods of education and evaluation. Recently evaluation has begun to focus on utility, practicality and improvement, and evaluators have begun to make recommendations based on their findings.

Conclusion

While the problem-based learning community has made some positive moves away from traditional quantitative-only evaluations of problem-based learning programmes, opportunities exist for further and future refinements. Mixed method reviews involving both qualitative and quantitative evaluation promise to provide depth and breadth to our analysis. Longitudinal studies can tell us whether problem-based learning is doing what we think it is by helping students learn deeply and retain information better. In the qualitative tradition, efforts to make meaning of multiple studies over time, similar to meta-analyses associated with the quantitative tradition, can help us make meaning of these qualitative evaluations so that they will perhaps be more transferable. These directions can provide programme evaluation with a positive future.

14

Sustaining problem-based learning curricula

Introduction

This chapter explores ways of sustaining problem-based learning curricula in terms of student motivation and curriculum development, and begins by examining the nature of problem-based learning curricula in the context of a learning community. We suggest that adopting some of the principles inherent in the development of learning communities is not only vital for the development of student identity, but also important for sustaining problem-based learning within universities. However, both the changing nature of learning in higher education and student motivation can affect the possibilities for sustaining problem-based learning communities. In the latter section of the chapter, we suggest central principles of curriculum review and reform that need to be taken into account to ensure the development and long-term sustainability of problem-based programmes.

Curricula as communities of practice?

One of the overarching principles of many problem-based learning curricula is the focus on learning as a shared responsibility, not only between students but also between tutors and students. This kind of acknowledgement, that no one individual is responsible for knowing everything, including the tutor, enables all those engaged in such a community to gain a sound understanding of both the content and process of learning. Such learning communities are seen as communities of practice where students are actively constructing understandings of what it means to be a professional. Lave and Wenger see learning

> not as a process of socially shared cognition that results in the end in the internalization of knowledge by individuals, but as a process of becoming a member of a sustained community of practice. Developing an

identity as a member of a community and becoming knowledgeably
skillful are part of the same process, with the former motivating, shaping
and giving meaning to the later, which it subsumes.

(Lave and Wenger 1991: 65)

Becoming a member of such a community involves developing knowledge
about the way it functions when she is a 'new comer' to it. Through the
learning process she first must come to understand the intuitive and explicit
practices of the community and then be able to participate in its socio-cultural
practices.

We suggest that using problem-based learning in programmes that are
educating students for the professions offers them an opportunity to begin
to develop understandings about their chosen profession's practices in ways
that are rarely possible in formal lecture-based programmes. Through the
problem-based learning team, they are able to test out knowledge as well as
construction of practice, guided by the facilitator, who in most cases will be a
member of that profession. In such a case, the facilitator would be classed, in
Lave and Wenger's (1991) terms, as an 'old timer' who will guide them
towards understandings of intuitive models of practice. Stronach *et al.* (2002)
have taken this a stage further and suggested that practice, while located
within a particular profession, relates more to the individuals within that
profession and their own 'ecologies of practice', such as experiences, beliefs
and practices that professionals accumulate in learning and performing
their roles. These ecologies relate largely to the kinds of knowledge that are
essentially intuitive or tacit and encompass particular ideologies that may be
personally held, but in the main are held by a particular profession.
Examples include ideals such as students needing to be inducted into a
profession through particular rituals and practices, ideologies about the
values of client-centred practice, the need for propositional knowledge as a
baseline for learning and convictions about the nature of good practice.

One of the main reasons that problem-based learning has become increasingly popular in education for the professions, and has been sustained over
time, is that the approach enables the promotion and sustaining of communities of practice. Certainly many facilitators have spoken of modelling
practice and inducting students into professional culture through problem-
based learning. Furthermore, the complexity of learning and working in
teams has been referred to as a means of mirroring practice. Many professionals are required to work in teams – teams that may not necessarily function effectively – and therefore tutors are keen to ensure that students learn
sound team skills, and are able to sustain teamwork while also developing in,
and with, the team. In Chapter 8 we suggested ways of preparing students to
work in teams, and it is important not only to prepare them but also to
ensure that both the level and quality of interaction is high and that assessment rewards collaboration as far as possible. Research by Lindblom-Ylänne
et al. (2003) explored student–student and tutor–student interaction in a
problem-based learning course in legal history. They examined study success

in relation to team dynamics and approaches to studying and noted that while there were differences between the three teams studied, one team achieved significantly higher grades. This was attributed to this team's students participating equally and more actively within the team setting than the students in the other two teams.

One of the important issues we have noted in problem-based learning teams is that although teams change and mature over time there are often key moments, *epiphanies*, when very significant changes occur in a team. An epiphany is when team members become excited, or make a new discovery, or suddenly start to make sense of something and become highly communicative. Sharing this new discovery with the team heightens team interaction and facilitates team progress. Denzin (1989) has proposed four different types of epiphanies. First, major epiphanies affect every part of an individual's life; he cites murder as a prime example. Second, a cumulative epiphany is where an individual experiences a turning point or reaction to events that have been occurring over a period of time, such as a woman experiencing domestic violence for years but deciding one day to leave the home. The third and fourth types are the ones we have seen in problem-based learning teams: the illuminative epiphany and the relived epiphany. The illuminative epiphany is where a problematic situation or issue suddenly becomes clear and the team or individual member is able to see how to resolve it. The relived epiphany is where the effect of an event is immediate, such as a bereavement, but meaning and sense-making only occur in reliving the event. So for example, in a problem-based learning team it is in reliving significant prior experiences that students may suddenly realize how to manage a situation facing them in a problem scenario.

We have found illuminative and relived epiphanies in evidence both in the stories of the students we interviewed (Savin-Baden 2000), and in the reflections of facilitators who have shared their experiences of watching teams make considerable shifts in their learning as a result of such epiphanies. Our research indicates that major shifts in teamwork and team functioning were almost always spoken of in relation to shifts (epiphanies) that radically altered and shaped the meanings that people gave to their learning in the team. Team epiphanies often occurred unexpectedly, were seen to be times of high creativity and were vital in terms of team development, progress and sustaining the team over time. However, in order to sustain such a vibrant learning community it is important that student interest and motivation to learn is maintained.

Sustaining student interest and motivation

Student motivation in higher education is currently an issue about which many tutors have concerns. The changing nature and purpose of higher education have led many to ask not only what higher education is for, but also what it *is* (for example, Barnett 1997, 2003). Higher education has changed globally since the 1980s, so there is now less emphasis on personal development and learning for its own sake. The university has become a place where knowledge is seen as a commodity (Barnett 1994: 13). Such changes have brought a shift in the notion of what it now means to be a strategic student. In the 1980s being strategic was largely seen as an intelligent approach to managing the system characterized by cue-seeking (Miller and Parlett 1974), through which students sought out cues in order to pass assessments. Entwistle (1981, 1987) suggested that a strategic approach to learning was characterized by an intention to obtain high grades, organize and distribute effort to greatest effect, use previous exam papers to predict questions and being alert to cues about marking schemes. More recently, strategic approaches have been characterized in terms of students who focus predominantly on social activities and part-time work, have little interest in their degree subject, have a poor attendance record and who tend not to submit work once a pass has been achieved (Kneale 1997). Kneale also points out that although the nature of teaching and learning in higher education is changing:

> What has not changed is the manner in which universities attempt to monitor, discipline and control student academic activities. There is still a background assumption that:
>
> (a) students want to be at university; and
> (b) students are interested in the degree subject they are studying.
>
> My view is that these two statements are less true than many colleagues think.
>
> (Kneale 1997: 119–20)

Higher education is increasingly becoming a place where knowledge is seen as a commodity and thus student motivation in undergraduate programmes is becoming an increasing concern to tutors. A study by Winn (2002) explored the impact of recent changes in the social and economic context of higher education on student motivation. She was able to categorize the students in the study into three types:

1   Those with demanding responsibilities and who did much academic work: these students had high employment or domestic commitments but managed to make a substantial commitment to their academic work simultaneously. These students were all highly motivated and went to great lengths to fit their studies into their busy lives.
2   Students with demanding personal lives but who did little academic work: this group had commitments in their personal lives that reduced the time available for academic work. Many of them found their daily lives highly stressful and this meant they felt they were unable to do more academic work. Many of these students put in more time around assessment deadlines as well as choosing not to do work that was not assessed.
3   Those with few responsibilities but who did little academic work: these students had no significant domestic or employment commitments and

most of them only did academic work that was assessed. These students adopted an instrumental approach to studying: they were motivated to pass their assessment and get a degree, but only by carrying out the minimum amount of work possible.

Winn suggested that there was potentially a fourth category of student: those with few responsibilities but who devoted much time to study. However, this group were not apparent in her study. The findings of this research suggest that harnessing students' enthusiasm for learning early in the course and helping them develop skills to become independent learners are a vital consideration for tutors. However, she suggests that such strategies will be limited in impact unless they are located within a government agenda that seeks to support those students who have responsibilities that impede their ability to study.

Thus it will be important that when problem-based learning is first implemented, strategies are adopted to ensure that student motivation is harnessed at the outset. It is also important that students are supported in adapting to problem-based learning when first encountering it as an approach to learning. Once they are accustomed to it, it is vital that their interest is both stimulated and maintained. For example, many course designers and problem-based tutors tend to follow a particular format to help novice students engage with the problem scenarios. Such a format enables students to understand how to begin to engage with the problem and also helps them to feel that they are supported in adapting to an approach to learning which may be unfamiliar to them. For example, it is common to adopt the seven steps to problem solving developed by University of Maastricht that are as follows:

1   Clarify and agree working definitions, unclear terms and concepts.
2   Define the problem and agree which phenomena require explanation.
3   Analyse the problems (brainstorm).
4   Arrange explanations into a tentative solution.
5   Generate and prioritize learning objectives.
6   Research the objectives through private study.
7   Report back, synthesize explanations and apply new information to the original problems.

Alternatively other tutors may use the form shown in Table 14.1 during the

Table 14.1 Establishing team learning needs

Ideas	Facts	Learning issues	Action plan

first seminar, which prompts students to think about their learning needs in terms of ideas and facts, and then to develop an action plan.

Although these strategies can be helpful to students new to problem-based learning, these steps can, over time, result in students becoming both rigid about using the format and formulaic in the way they tackle the problem. The result is then that students become apathetic towards problem-based learning because it is no longer a creative process. Similarly, if there is insufficient variety in the type of problems used, students may also become disenchanted. For example, a nursing programme we were involved with, despite our early advice, used triggers based largely on paper cases in the first two years of the programme with very little other type of scenario. Students began to complain that the problems were very much the same. When we analysed the problems we saw that they did differ in type and complexity, but the format used and the way they were presented had many similarities. The problems were then adapted to include different kinds of audio and visual stimuli: storyboards, video clips, card games, voicemail messages and laboratory results, and this has promoted greater interest for both tutors and students.

However, it is not only the types of students within the university and the nature of problems that demand attention, but also the issues connected to the way in which problem-based learning has been placed into the existing curriculum. There is often a tendency to believe that, if considerable time and effort is spent in designing and implementing a problem-based learning programme, thereafter it will merely require minimal tweaking here and there. This is not the case. Problem-based programmes that eventually dissolve do so largely because those involved have not engaged with some or all of the issues regarding curriculum review and reform that we suggest below.

Curriculum review and reform

As we noted in Chapter 4, there are many ways in which it is possible to implement problem-based learning. However, since some programmes have been in existence for more than 20 years, there are concerns about the changes that are experienced over time in such programmes, how they are sustained and reformed, and the extent to which they move away from the original aims of the programme.

A recent series of articles has debated the place of basic sciences in medical curricula that used problem-based learning. Glew (2003) began by arguing that although the implementation of problem-based learning in medical education was well founded, the way in which it had been implemented had compromised its potential. However, White (2003) suggested that Glew's disillusionment with the approach was not caused by its implementation, but by three particular difficulties. These were, poor support from basic scientists who did not embrace problem-based learning, poor oversight by the administration charged with implementing problem-based learning, and over-reliance on clinical educators who were unmotivated or insufficiently knowledgeable to teach basic science. Therefore, little of what was being argued over could particularly be blamed on the learning approach. Instead, the difficulties seemed to be emerging from a number of issues that can be generalized to many curricula that utilize problem-based learning, which include:

- the role and perception of the facilitator, present or otherwise;
- the way problem-based learning is implemented in the curriculum;
- the unplanned-for long-term running cost of problem-based learning;
- the extent to which facilitators experience burn out;
- the way in which tutors are trained, equipped and updated;
- the extent to which assessment is driving the learning;
- a debate about whether learning through problem-based learning is different, depending upon the discipline;
- the extent to which 'curricula drift' occurs within the first two years of a programme.

While we have addressed many of these issues in other areas of this text we return to them here briefly as they are important for sustaining and reforming problem-based curricula.

The way problem-based learning is implemented in the curriculum

We discussed in Chapter 4 that it is possible to implement problem-based learning in one module or across a whole curriculum. We have also argued elsewhere (Savin-Baden 2000) that the particular models of problem-based learning adopted and the different emphases on knowledge, assessment and the roles taken by both the students and the facilitator will affect the kinds of learning opportunities on offer to students. However, the way it is implemented and the personal and institutional costs will also affect the extent to which it is possible to sustain problem-based learning.

The unplanned-for long-term running cost of problem-based learning

We have had several discussions with zealous tutors who have begun implementing problem-based learning but soon found they were unable to sustain it in more than one or two courses. For example, a scientist in one university explained how the tutors who were keen to implement problem-based learning used all their allocated teaching time on developing and sustaining problem-based learning in the first year of a programme. The first year of the programme was very successful and the student feedback was excellent. The difficulty was that few other tutors in this department were interested in taking up problem-based learning, and the tutors who had offered a superb first year were struggling to be able to offer the same standard and quality in the second year because of their first-year teaching commitments. It is important at the outset to consider resources and personal and institutional costs in terms of implementation and sustaining the programme.

Facilitator burn-out

Over the last few years there has been an ongoing discussion about what has been termed 'facilitator burn-out' or 'facilitator fatigue'. To date there has been little, if any, research into this but what is being described is a position where problem-based learning facilitators have become tired, bored and dissatisfied with facilitation. There would seem to be a number of ways of dealing with this. The first is that when implementing problem-based learning initially it is important to plan an educational development programme for as many tutors as possible, but not to use them all as facilitators at the outset. Ideally, facilitators should be involved with problem-based learning for a period of three years and then spend at least a year away from problem-based learning, by teaching on other parts of the programme, doing research or taking on a more administrative role. Few problem-based programmes use this approach exclusively and many choose to use lectures, skills sessions, fieldwork and other approaches in order to provide diversity for students. Facilitator burn-out would seem to occur most in tutors who value and enjoy problem-based learning and who, because other tutors refuse to get involved, often facilitate too many teams or feel they have to do more problem-based learning than anything else.

Training, equipping and updating facilitators

Although we discuss ways of providing initial and ongoing training and development for problem-based learning facilitators in detail in Chapter 10, we also raise it here, as we believe it is an issue that is important for sustaining curricula. The increase in the use of problem-based learning has brought with it a great demand for tutor and educational development. In some disciplines and countries the focus is on tutor development, in others it is on educational development. Tutor development in general tends to focus upon equipping tutors with skills to implement problem-based learning through training workshops that offer hints and tips. This may comprise a series of training days on given topics such as trigger development, assessment, small group learning and how to use problem-based learning in large groups. The difficulty with tutor development programmes that are essentially 'how to' training sessions is that they begin with the assumption that participants just need a few particular skills that could simply be applied categorically across all subjects and disciplines, with little thought to the discipline itself or to the constructivist nature of problem-based learning.

Tutor development that comprises training in *techniques* is not needed; what is required instead is educational development so that tutors are encouraged to review their position in an educational way. In practice the workshop should not contain hints and tips, but should engage tutors with problem-based learning by first exploring the concept of the curriculum and the place of this approach within it. This emphasis helps tutors not only to examine their assumptions about what might count as a curriculum, but also to explore their understandings about learning and knowledge, and their views about autonomy, authority and control. This will mean that instead of just tutoring problem-based learning, tutors will become active in improving, developing and sustaining their programme.

The extent to which assessment is driving learning

Often in discussions with tutors, we find that it is not the nature of assessment that people are worrying about but student failure. Students who fail complain, give us bad feedback, and sob quietly as we try to console them. Yet if our systems were different perhaps tutors and students would begin to see failure as part of the developmental process of learning, rather than as a differentiation between those who *can* and those who *cannot*. In Chapter 12, we have suggested ways of changing assessment to fit better with problem-based learning, but many of the forms of assessment that we still use are bounded by our need to stratify students and thus this defines the learning of an individual student as something that is or is not valuable. What we need to focus on instead is the development of learning power, which Claxton (2000) has suggested is 'getting better at knowing when, how and what to do when you don't know what to do'. For many of us, assessment is part of the learning and is designed to help students progress to another (higher) level of learning, yet we often find it hard to make this explicit or find ways of enabling students to see assessment as part of their learning journey. For them assessment is often about being strategic, cue conscious, and decoding what is really required. Harris (2001) has suggested that plagiarism often occurs because students do not understand what is required of them in assessment, and has argued that tutors need to make both the intentions and the language used in assessment clear to students. We believe that this is vital in problem-based learning, particularly when peer assessment is being used. Assessment appears to be a major pitfall in sustaining problem-based learning because the approach demands that we ensure that there is alignment between what students are learning (as opposed to being taught) and the assessment.

The extent to which learning through problem-based learning is different depending upon the discipline

The rules and codes that bind disciplines and affect what is deemed to be acceptable have given rise to discussion about tribes and territories (Becher and Trowler 2001). Other authors have suggested, for example, that 'the culture of the discipline includes idols: the pictures on the walls and dust jackets of books kept in view are of Albert Einstein and Max Planck and Robert Oppenheimer in the office of the physicist and of Max Weber and Karl Marx and Emile Durkheim in the office of the sociologist' (Clark 1980: 4). There is still a sense that problem-based learning can largely look the same and be utilized the same way across most disciplines. Yet the disciplinary differences do have an impact on problem-based learning because it is affected by the codes of the discipline. For example, what it means to pose an argument, write an essay, or put a case forward will differ whether you are teaching English, law, medicine or golf. It is important to consider what the impact of using problem-based learning will be upon disciplinary codes and vice versa, when seeking to implement and sustain the approach over time.

Curricula drift

The idea of curricula drift is that over a relatively short period of time (2–5 years) a problem-based learning programme drifts away from its original foundations and becomes a diluted version. This often occurs because individual tutors refuse to change their pedagogical approach to learning because they do not see the value of problem-based learning. Alternatively, tutors may feel that by allowing students a greater degree of autonomy than in former years that they no longer have control over what is learnt. For other tutors this may occur because fundamentally they do not believe that their areas of the programme can be best taught through problem-based learning and therefore they use problem-based learning tutorials as lecture slots. This last issue has tended to occur particularly in the area of teaching basic science to students. For example, Jones *et al.* (2001) note that at the University of Washington curricular drift occurred after five years 'with both basic scientists and clinicians showing regression to the mean in terms of reintroducing and teaching topics, and expanding teaching times, partly in response to financial pressure' (Jones *et al.* 2001: 701). Preventing curricula drift can be addressed through long-term tutor development and by ensuring that the approach is closely monitored and evaluated.

Conclusion

Sustaining problem-based learning courses, modules and programmes is a demanding and complex business. Recognizing that such programmes are communities of practice can help tutors and students realize the importance of the shared responsibility for maintaining them through questioning, critique and feedback. Nevertheless, the changing nature of higher education and the position of problem-based learning within the curriculum have a strong influence on the possibility for maintaining the approach in the long term. What is important is that administrators and tutors recognize the need for long-term tutor development, the possibility of facilitator burn-out, the impact of disciplinary difference, and that problem-based learning is implemented in ways that are both realistic and sustainable.

Epilogue: future imperative?

Introduction

Throughout this text we have explored theories of learning that relate to problem-based learning and issues connected to curriculum and problem design, examined the role of tutors and students, debated issues of culture and diversity and explored ways of sustaining problem-based curricula. Yet where should the community go from here? What are the real issues connected with moving ourselves as tutors, our institutions and the problem-based learning community forward in terms of research, teaching and action relating to problem-based learning? In this final section of the book we raise areas that we feel need to be addressed in the years ahead. They include online learning and problem-based learning, the complexities of promoting collaborative learning and the impact of ideas such as graduateness and employability on problem-based learning. We begin first by examining problem-based learning and online learning.

Online problem-based learning: a virtual fantasy?

The term 'computer-mediated problem-based learning' has been used initially to define any form of problem-based learning that utilizes computers in some way. However, this is problematic since it offers little indication about the ways in which computers are being used, the areas of interaction of the students, the quality of the learning materials or the extent to which any of these fit with problem-based learning. Many virtual learning environments such as WebCT and Blackboard are being used in universities, yet most are little more than information repositories for lecture notes, because the university managers have issued a directive that 'everything that is vital for a student to know must be on WebCT'. This raises questions about what it is that is vital for students to know, and whether the virtual lecturing notes are helpful in support of this knowing. Furthermore, there are other issues that need to be taken into account, such as developing tutors' online facilitation capabilities, providing some synchronous events to support students, encouraging collaborative interactive participation and finding ways of engaging students who seldom participate in the online problem-based learning team.

Electronic learning, of whatever sort, needs to be pedagogically informed and if it is being used to support problem-based learning it needs to be well designed to ensure that the weaknesses of both approaches are addressed. Thus we suggest that computer-mediated collaborative problem-based learning needs to be focused on a team-orientated knowledge building discourse and that students should work collaboratively in real-time or asynchronously to manage the problem. Although using online learning in conjunction with problem-based learning has a number of advantages, such as students having access to wider resources and often innovative problems (see, for example, the Students Online in Nursing Integrated Curricula Project 2003), new and different forms of dialogue and immediacy in learning and communication, there are also a number of disadvantages. For example, students can be overloaded with information and the problem scenarios may be all at the same level, with gradients being seen in terms of complexity of information management rather than of the development of criticality. Computer-mediated collaborative problem-based learning can also result in communication problems both within the team and between team and facilitator, because of the difficulties of understanding text-talk rather than real talk. Problem-based learning is an approach that relies strongly on communication and learning through dialogue, and if communication through text messaging or e-mail is misunderstood or tutor feedback is seen as negative by the team when it is not meant to be, this can lead to confusion and disjunction. In many ways it could be argued that designing computer-mediated collaborative problem-based learning programmes is no different from other forms of problem-based learning, in that it needs to be designed with sound pedagogical foundations and not as a means of either solving other curricula difficulties such as too many students and too much information or merely providing an innovative approach to learning.

Promoting collaborative learning

One of the central principles of problem-based learning is that students work and learn in teams. The size of the team varies depending on the discipline, cohort and university but the general trend in the UK is to utilize teams of 8–12 students and in the USA teams of around 6 members. Yet in our fragmented and incoherent society there are difficulties with commitment and teamwork. Discussions in the press and over dinner at conferences often centre on what it means to be a student at university, for example, 'Are they there to read for a degree? Does supplying handouts to facilitate learning constitute the promotion of a dependency culture in higher education?' In problem-based learning the questions about what counts as attendance and how students can be encouraged to be committed to the team, but also be autonomous learners, is still hotly debated.

Many of the texts on groups and teamwork have argued that team members should help to develop conditions where each member can negotiate, cooperate and fulfil their own needs. In the context of problem-based learning two principles in particular can help teams to develop such conditions. First, exploring the principle of autonomy means that students have freedom to choose, take decisions and then be accountable for such decisions. This principle also means that facilitators must honour the right of the students to make choices about what they do and do not do in the team, and an informed choice about activities in which they will be expected to participate. Such a principle is a good one, but in the context of higher education and current models of problem-based learning this is difficult to implement. Part of the challenge here is because of the second principle: that of informed consent. There are a number of difficulties with informed consent. For example, different types of consent have different implications for the team and the curriculum as a whole. Much of the consent that occurs in teaching and particularly problem-based learning is either tacit consent, agreement through not objecting or implied consent, which is inferred from actions. Thus commitment to the team and what staff and students mean by commitment is complex and often remains uncontested by students. The result is that sometimes students fall short of commitment to the team, but the conflict that often ensues is invariably ignored and dealt with neither by the team nor the facilitator.

The challenge for many problem-based facilitators is to encourage and sustain the principles of autonomy and informed consent in the context of assessment, competition and demanding workloads. It is often the case that difficulties in relationships between students and their facilitator and among team members themselves are caused to some extent by the idea of having an implicit understanding of trust and non-concealment. Trust in teams is fragile and something that needs to be built, maintained and sustained. Honesty in teams is often difficult with high workloads, endless assessment deadlines, normally caused by modularization, and the temptation to plagiarize. Thus ethical questions do not rest purely around the issues about how to behave – ethics have to be understood in terms of the relationships made with those in the team. This can be particularly difficult for facilitators since some situations are problematic, because they place the facilitator in a position where her obligations as a facilitator conflict with those as a tutor in higher education.

Individualism is both prevalent and promoted in most cultures worldwide and this is causing difficulties for team-based learning approaches. The perception of students as consumers seems to be promoting a notion of individualism that signals an end to dialogue and with it a devaluing of collaborative and dialogic approaches to learning. Yet we would suggest that transactional dialogue (after Brookfield 1985), where the team serves as an interactive function for the individual, is vital for maintaining and sustaining problem-based learning teams. Such a focus will mean that individual students, by making themselves and their learning the focus of reflection and analysis within the team, are able to value alternative ways of knowing. Dialogue thus becomes central to progress both in the students' and the team's lives and it is through dialogue that values are deconstructed and reconstructed, and experiences relived and explored, in order to make sense of roles and relationships. It is only by engaging with students in debates about dialogic learning, individualism and the impact of wider political concerns on their learning that we can begin to help our students to take a stance towards knowledge and encourage them to become critical beings.

Employability and graduateness: political ends for problem-based learning?

Employability and graduateness have been a focus in higher education for many years but it would seem that more recently, these areas have increasingly become the centre of political attention. Problem-based learning is increasingly being used as a means of supporting and promoting the idea of graduateness. The term 'graduateness' is now being used worldwide to describe particular generic skills and qualities that graduates are seen to possess. Barrie (2003) has explored the rhetoric of generic graduate attributes and shown that Australian academics 'do not share a common understanding of either the nature of these outcomes or the teaching and learning processes that might facilitate the development of these outcomes' (Barrie 2003: 1). Such findings would seem to indicate that academics who lay claim to the development of generic capabilities are more likely to espouse the rhetoric than the reality. However, what is not entirely clear is how it is possible to identify the development of these attributes in learning contexts and whether it is possible to argue that particular approaches to learning (or even disciplines) put more or less emphasis on different attributes. For example, some tutors may argue that problem-based learning promotes problem-solving as an attribute that is transferable to the workplace, but to date there is little evidence to support this. Yet there is still a growing concern that graduates do not have attributes that employers expect.

Employability is largely seen as employers' expectations of what graduates can supply when they first arrive at the workplace. These expectations are usually formulated in terms of particular skills or competences that may include problem-solving skills, self-management skills and communication skills. The reality in the past is that not only have these skills been seen as instrumental and transferable, but also as outcomes that can be attributed to particular curricula or forms of learning. Such understandings have meant that skills have been downgraded as something basic, instead of being seen as complex capabilities that take time to develop, and are often tacit and difficult to define. Thus, although employers may feel that they can list the skills they require of graduates, actually what most of them really require are complex capabilities. Are notions of employability actually about the development of skills? We think not. However complex the skills are seen to be, we would argue that what employers really want are 'learning capabilities'. Such capabilities would include reflexivity, meta analysis, problem-management, tacit understanding and meta leadership, to name just a few. These are not basic skills but complex capabilities that have emerged through learning that is not about swallowing chunks of knowledge but about learning with complexity and through transactional dialogue. We would suggest that these capabilities are not just what employers want but what we would see as qualities of 'graduateness'. Such capabilities can be learnt and honed through forms of problem-based learning that promote contestability and enable students to develop a critical position from which to interpret the practice of others. However, to argue for the implementation of problem-based learning with the justification that it will necessarily ensure the development of graduate attributes and employability is certainly dangerous ground.

Retrospect and prospect

Problem-based learning in and for the future needs to be seen as an approach to learning that is not just about employability, widening access, using new technologies or as the 'happening' new *genre* in higher education learning. It needs to be seen as an approach to learning that really does help students to engage *with* and live *in* a complex world.

   Much of this text has explored principles and issues that need to be considered when implementing problem-based learning. It has also been a text that has raised questions about problem-based learning as an approach, a community and as a mode of curriculum practice. Thus we hope that it has not only provided some foundations for those tutors new or relatively new to problem-based learning, but also interrupted some thoughts and provided some arguments for those experienced in this field. It would seem that problem-based learning, while here to stay, is and will remain contested ground. The pure models are dead and cannot be resurrected or redeemed in our postmodern world. New ideologies and practices have emerged – all we have to do is decide how we position ourselves in relation to them.

Appendix

Methods of assessment for problem-based learning

The following section lists some of the forms of assessment that have been used successfully with problem-based learning and which also allow movement away from the need to have outcome-based examinations.

Group presentation

Asking the students to submit their work orally or in written form as a collaborative piece models the process of problem-based learning but is difficult to mark. Is content, process, presentation or a combination of these being marked?

Individual presentation

Here students are asked to submit the component of work that they have researched for their contribution to the overall solution or management of the problem scenario. This has some of the problems of the above and if the students just present the component they have researched there is little synthesis overall with the problem scenario. This is also time-consuming with large cohorts.

Tripartite assessment

This has three components:

1 The group submits a report for which they receive a mark.
2 The individual submits the piece of work they researched.
3 The individual writes an account of the team process that is linked to the theory of small group work.

These three components are added together to form the overall individual mark. The advantage of this is that it does not privilege any students who do less work and each individual student will be responsible for gaining two-thirds of their own mark, so that most students perceive this kind of grading as being fair.

Case-based individual essay

Here the student is presented with a case scenario that they respond to in the form of an essay. Students may be given a choice of scenarios from which to choose and the level of detail and complexity can vary from year to year. This links well with problem-based learning but still tends to focus largely on cognitive abilities (unless students are allowed to use narrative style essays).

Case-based care plan based in clinical practice/client-led project

Here students are presented with a real life scenario to solve/manage for a client. One group of engineering students were given a bunch of coconuts and asked to design an effective tool to remove both the flesh and the milk. Another set of students were asked to resolve the difficulty of cracks occurring in railway lines crossing Central Australia caused by the excessive heat and train vibration. These are very effective but must be criterion-referenced and are, therefore, disliked by some tutors and external examiners if the criteria are perceived to be too broad.

Portfolios

These can be unwieldy if not managed well and are difficult to mark, but they are fine if they are well designed. Portfolios have been used in a number of programmes that educate students for the professions. In recent years the requirements for these have been refined away from a vast quantity of materials towards a slenderer version that offers greater reflection and critic-ality than before. Attention must be paid to marking criteria to ensure there is a requirement to create an overall synthesis.

Triple jump (Painvin *et al.* 1979; Powles *et al.* 1981)

Here individual students are presented with a problem and expected to discuss the problem and their learning needs with an oral examiner. Students then locate relevant material and later discuss their findings with the examiner and are rated on problem-solving skills, self-directed learning skills, and on their knowledge of the problem area. This is an assessment that has been specifically developed for problem-based learning, but it is time consuming and costly and tends only to be used in well-funded programmes with small student numbers.

Viva voce examinations

These were used very effectively before problem-based learning became popular and have since been adopted by several curriculum designers for use with problem-based learning. However, they are best done in practice situations and although very effective, can be costly, time consuming and extremely stressful for the student.

Reflective (online) journals

These have worked well in engineering and health. Students hand them in each week and receive a mark at the end of each term/semester. Students tend to be more open and honest about their learning than one would expect and these can be criterion-referenced.

Reports

Written communication is an important skill for students to acquire. Requiring written reports allows students to practise this form of communication, particularly if the word allowance is short and it is used in the final year, as it can promote succinct, critical pieces of work.

Patchwork text (Winter *et al.* 1999)

This is a way of getting students to present their work in written form. Students build up text in coursework over a number of weeks. Each component of work is shared with other students and they are expected to use different styles, such as a commentary on a lecture, a personal account or a book review. This kind of assessment fits well with problem-based learning because of its emphasis on critique and self-questioning.

Self-assessment

This works well with problem-based learning, but students must be equipped to undertake it. Self-assessment allows students to think more carefully about what they do and do not know, and what they additionally need to know to accomplish certain tasks. Confusion arises in many courses in understanding the difference between self, peer and collaborative assessment (but we discuss this below). It involves students judging their own work. It may include essays, presentations, reports and reflective diaries. One of the difficulties with self-assessment is the tendency to make judgements about what the students meant rather than what they actually achieved. Boud has defined self-assessment as: 'The involvement of students in identifying standards and/or criteria to apply to their work and making judgments about the extent to which they have met these criteria and standards' (Boud 1986: 12).

Collaborative assessment

The student assesses her/himself in light of the criteria agreed with the tutor. The tutor assesses the student using the same criteria and they negotiate a final grade.

Peer assessment

A good fit with problem-based learning. It involves students making judgements about other students' work, either by using their own assessment criteria or that provided by tutors, which can sometimes be better. This kind of assessment also emphasizes the cooperative nature of the problem-based learning environment. It is generally used for presentations and practical examinations but it can also be used for essays and exam scripts. Using peer assessment with essays is really useful with problem-based learning and also highly informative for student and tutor. It can be carried out in a variety of ways including:

- anonymously with assessors randomly chosen,
- openly but with several assessors used to assess each element of the work.

Inter-peer assessment
This is where students from one problem-based learning team assess the work of another team.

Intra-peer assessment
Students assess the product of what they themselves have produced as a team.

Self- and peer assessment in problem-based learning have both advantages and disadvantages:

1   As a result of peer and self-assessment many students perform better on other forms of assessment.
2   It encourages students to move away from strategic approaches to learning.
3   It encourages honesty and personal responsibility in the team.
4   It promotes the valuing of the process of learning.
5   Problems occur if external examiners are not experienced in self- and peer assessment and are consequently suspicious of its reliability or validity.
6   There is a tendency for some tutors and students still to think in terms of norm rather than criterion-referenced marking and judging performance against that of others rather than on its own merits.
7   It can be time consuming to set up.
8   Tutors often feel they need to moderate self- and peer assessment.
9   Our higher education systems do not support self- and peer assessment because they largely reward students with individual grades.
10 Many tutors are confused about the difference between collaborative, peer and self-assessment and use the terms together or interchangeably.

Glossary

Collaborative assessment – where the student assesses her/himself in light of the criteria agreed with the tutor. The tutor assesses the student using the same criteria and they negotiate a final grade.

Complexity skills – the advanced skills which go beyond key skills and subject skills in a qualification framework, such as the capacity to work in complex and ambiguous contexts and to solve and manage problems in ways that transcend conventional lines of thinking.

Critical contestability – a position whereby students understand and acknowledge the transient nature of subject and discipline boundaries. They are able to transcend and interrogate these boundaries through a commitment to exploring the subtext of subjects and disciplines.

Descriptive knowledge – knowledge that comprises empirical facts. Such knowledge describes the fact of a situation. For example, aspirin reduces the chance of a heart attack occurring.

Declarative knowledge – knowledge of the world as it is; essentially the same as propositional knowledge.

Dialogic learning – learning that occurs when insights and understandings emerge through dialogue in a learning environment. It is a form of learning where students draw upon their own experience to explain the concepts and ideas with which they are presented, and then use that experience to make sense for themselves and also to explore further issues.

Disjunction – a sense of fragmentation of part of, or all of the self, characterized by frustration and confusion, and a loss of sense of self, which often results in anger and the need for right answers.

Domain – the overlapping spheres within a stance. The borders of the domains merge with one another and therefore shifts between domains are transitional areas where particular kinds of learning occur.

Explanatory knowledge – knowledge of causal theories, knowledge that explains something. This kind of knowledge would explain why aspirin reduces the chances of developing a heart attack.

Facilitator – the tutor/faculty/member of staff who enables learning to take place in the context of problem-based learning.

Feedback session – the session where students feedback to the problem-based learning team the information they have discovered individually which relates to the problem scenario.

Frame factors – issues that are raised by the students that do not directly relate to the problem scenario. For example, transport between campuses, the arrival of student uniforms or students' personal problems.

Interactional stance – the ways in which learners work and learn in teams and construct meaning in relation to one another.

Inter-peer assessment – this is where students from a problem-based learning team assess the work of another team.

Interprofessional education – the use of a variety of teaching methods and learning strategies to encourage interaction and interactive learning across the professions which includes the development of skills and attitudes as well as knowledge.

Intra-peer assessment – students assess the product of what they themselves have produced as a team.

Introductory session – the first problem-based learning session where the problem scenario is presented to the students.

Key skills – skills such as working with others, problem solving and improving personal learning and performance that it is expected would be required of students in the world of work.

Learner identity – an identity formulated through the interaction of learner and learning. The notion of learner identity moves beyond, but encapsulates the notion of learning style, and encompasses positions that students take up in learning situations, whether consciously or unconsciously.

Learning context – the interplay of all the values, beliefs, relationships, frameworks and external structures that operate within a given learning environment.

Learning in relation – the ways in which students learn with and through others in such ways that they are helped to make connections between their lives, with other subjects and disciplines and with personal concerns. Learning in relation also incorporates not only the idea that students learn, as it were, in relation to their own knowledge and experience, but also to that of others.

Mode 1 knowledge (Gibbons *et al.* 1994) – propositional knowledge that is produced within the academe separate from its use. Academe is considered the traditional environment for the generation of Mode 1 knowledge.

Mode 2 knowledge (Gibbons *et al.* 1994) – this knowledge transcends disciplines and is produced in and validated through the world of work. Knowing in this mode demands the integration of skills and abilities in order to act in a particular context.

Peer assessment – involves students making judgements about other students' work. Ideally the students design their own assessment criteria and use them to assess each other, but in many programmes they are designed by tutors.

Pedagogical stance – the ways in which people see themselves as learners in particular educational environments.

Performative slide – the increasing focus in higher education on what students are able to *do*, which has emerged from the desire to equip students for life and work. Higher education is sliding towards encouraging students to perform rather than to necessarily critique and do.

Personal knowledge – knowledge about oneself and one's perspectives on the world, as represented through attitudes and convictions. Such knowledge is acquired through culture, class and experience.

Personal stance – the way in which tutors and students see themselves in relation to the learning context and give their own distinctive meaning to their experience of that context.

Problem-based learning team – a number of students who work together as a defined group.

Problem-solving learning – teaching where the focus is on students solving a given problem by acquiring the answers expected by the tutor, answers that are rooted in the information supplied in some way to the students. The solutions are bounded by the content and students are expected to explore little extra material other than that provided, in order to discover the solutions.

Procedural knowledge – knowledge of how to act in a situation in order to change it.

Propositional knowledge – the kind of knowledge that for some time has been seen as that which includes discipline-based theories and concepts derived from bodies of knowledge, practical principles and generalizations, and specific propositions about particular cases, decisions or actions.

Self-assessment – this involves students developing standards to apply to their work and making judgements about the extent to which they have met these criteria.

Stance – one's attitude, belief or disposition towards a particular context, person or experience. It refers to a particular position one takes up in life towards something, at a particular point in time.

Team – a group of people who work together with a common purpose. There is a limited membership and the team has the power to make decisions. Teams have a focus, a set of team rules, and are time limited.

Tutor – a member of the teaching staff in the university, usually denoted as 'staff' in the UK and as 'faculty' in the USA.

Transition – shifts in learner experience caused by a challenge to the person's life-world. Transitions occur in particular areas of students' lives, at different times and in distinct ways. The notion of transitions carries with it the idea of movement from one place to another and with it the necessity of taking up a new position in a different place.

Transitional learning – learning that occurs as a result of critical reflection upon shifts (transitions) that have taken place for the students personally (including viscerally), pedagogically and/or interactionally.

Bibliography

Ahn, D. (1999) Visiting elective students at the University of Toronto from the Korea University Medical College, *Medical Education*, 33: 460–5.

Albanese, M.A. and Mitchell, S. (1993) Problem-based learning: A review of literature on its outcomes and implementation issues, *Academic Medicine*, 68(1): 52–68.

Allen, J.S. and Coulson, R. (2000) A problem-based, self-learning core curriculum at Southern Illinois University Carbondale: A proposal to the William and Flora Hewlett Foundation. http://mccoy.lib.siu.edu/corecurr/pbl/acrobats/ proposal. pdf (accessed 10 September 2003).

Almy, T.P., Colby, K.K., Zubkoff, M., Gephart, D.S., Moore-West, M. and Lundquist, L.L. (1992) Health, society, and the physician: Problem-based learning of the social sciences and humanities, *Annals of Internal Medicine*, 116(7): 569–74.

Andersen, B. and McMillan, M. (1991) Learning experiences for professional reality and responsibility. Paper presented to National Experiential Learning Conference. University of Surrey, 16–18 July.

Anderson, R. (1998) Why talk about different ways to grade? The shift from traditional assessment to alternative assessment, *New Directions for Teaching and Learning*, 74: 5–16.

Anderson, R.C. (1984) Role of the reader's schema in comprehension, learning, and memory, in R.C. Anderson, J. Osborn and R.J. Tierney (eds) *Learning to read in American schools: Basal readers and content texts*. Hillsdale, NJ: Lawrence Erlbaum.

Angelo, T.A. (1995) Assessing (and defining) assessment, *The AAHE Bulletin*, 48(3): 7.

Ashworth, P.J. (2003) Developing usable pedagogic research skills. Keynote speech presented to the 11th Improving Student Learning Symposium. Improving Student Learning: Theory Research and Scholarship. Hinckley, UK, 1–3 September.

Astin, A.W. (1993) *What Matters in College: Four Critical Years Revisited*. San Francisco, Jossey-Bass.

Astin, A.W., Banta, T.W., Cross, K.P., El-Khawas, E., Ewell, P.T., Hutchings, P., Marchese, T.J., McClenney, K.M., Mentkowski, M., Miller, M.A., Moran, E.T. and Wright, B.D., (n.d.) *Assessment Forum: 9 Principles of Good Practice for Assessing Student Learning*. Washington, DC: American Association for Higher Education.

Ausubel, D.P., Novak, J.S. and Hanesian, H. (1978) *Educational Psychology: A Cognitive View*. New York: Holt, Rinehart and Winston.

Barnett, R. (1994) *The Limits of Competence*. Buckingham: SRHE/Open University Press.

Barnett, R. (1997) *Higher Education: A Critical Business*. Buckingham: SRHE/Open University Press.

Barnett, R. (2000) *Realizing the University in an Age of Supercomplexity*. Buckingham: SRHE/Open University Press.

Barnett, R. (2001) 'Evidence-based practice': a sceptic's view. Keynote Speech to the 2nd International Conference on Qualitative Evidence-based Practice, Coventry University, May 14–16.

Barnett, R. (2003) *Beyond all Reason: Living with Ideology in the University*. Buckingham: SRHE/Open University Press.

Barnett, R. and Coates, K. (2002) *Conceptualizing Curricula: A Schema. Imaginative Curriculum Knowledge Development Paper 2*. April. LTSN Generic Centre www.ltsn.ac.uk/genericcentre (accessed 20 May 2002).

Barr, R.B. and Tagg, J. (1995) From teaching to learning – a new paradigm for undergraduate education, *Change Magazine*, 27(6): 12–25.

Barrie, S. (2003) Using conceptions of graduate attributes for research-led systematic curriculum reform. Paper presented to the 11th Improving Student Learning Symposium. Improving Student Learning: Theory Research and Scholarship. Hinckley, UK, 1–3 September.

Barrows, H.S. (1986) A taxonomy of problem-based learning methods, *Medical Education*, 20: 481–6.

Barrows, H.S. (1988) *The Tutorial Process*. Springfield Illinois: Southern Illinois University School of Medicine.

Barrows, H.S. (2000) *Problem-Based Learning Applied to Medical Education*. Springfield, Illinois: Southern Illinois University School of Medicine.

Barrows, H.S. and Bennett, K. (1972) Experimental studies on the diagnostic (problem-solving) skill of the neurologist, their implications for neurological training, *Archives of Neurology*, 26: 273–7.

Barrows, H.S. and Tamblyn, R. (1976) An evaluation of problem-based learning in small groups utilizing a simulated patient, *Journal of Medical Education*, 51(1): 52–4.

Barrows, H.S. and Tamblyn, R. (1977) The portable patient problem pack: A problem-based learning unit, *Journal of Medical Education*, 52(12): 1002–4.

Barrows, H.S. and Tamblyn, R.M. (1980) *Problem-Based Learning: An Approach to Medical Education*. New York: Springer.

Baume, D. and Baume, C. (1994) Staff and educational development: a discussion paper, *SEDA Newsletter*, 2 (March) 6–9.

Becher, T. and Trowler, P.R. (2001) *Academic Tribes and Territories*, 2nd edn. Buckingham: SRHE/Open University Press.

Becker, H. (1970) Whose side are we on?, in J.D. Douglas (ed.) *The Relevance of Sociology*. New York: Appleton-Century Crofts.

Belbin, R.M. (1993) *Team Roles at Work*. Oxford: Butterworth Heinemann.

Belenky, M.F., Clinchy, B.M., Goldberger, N.R. and Tarule, J.M. (1986) *Women's Ways of Knowing*. New York: Basic Books Inc.

Berkson, L. (1993) Problem-based learning: Have expectations been met? *Academic Medicine*, 68: 579–88 (October supplement).

Bernstein, B. (1992) Pedagogic identities and educational reform. Paper given to Santiago conference, Cepal, 11 November, mimeo.

Bernstein, P., Tipping, J., Bercovitz, K. and Skinner, H.A. (1995) Shifting students and faculty to a PBL curriculum: attitudes changed and lessons learned. *Academic Medicine*, 70: 245–7.

Biggs, J. (1997) Teaching across and within cultures: the issue of international students, in R. Murray-Harvey and H.C. Silins (eds) *Learning and Teaching in Higher Education: Advancing International Perspectives, Proceedings of the Higher Education Research and Development Society of Australasia Conference*, Adelaide: Higher Education Research and Development Society of Australasia, 1–22.

Biggs, J. (1999) *Teaching for Quality Learning at University*. Buckingham: SRHE/Open University Press.

Bloom, B. (1956) *Taxonomy of Educational Objectives*, 2 vols. New York: Longmans Green.

Blumberg, P. and Michael, J.A. (1992) Development of self-directed learning behaviors in a partially teacher-directed problem-based learning curriculum, *Teaching and Learning in Medicine*, 4(1): 3–8.

Bosworth, K. (1994) Developing Collaborative Skills in College Students Collaborative Learning: Underlying Processes and Effective Techniques, in K. Bosworth and S.J. Hamilton (eds) *New Directions for Teaching and Learning*, No. 59. San Francisco: Jossey-Bass, pp. 25–31.

Boud, D. (ed.) (1985) *Problem-based Learning in Education for the Professions*. Sydney: Higher Education Research and Development Society of Australasia.

Boud, D. (1986) *Implementing Student Self-Assessment*. HERDSA Green Guide, No. 5. Sydney: Higher Education Research and Development Society of Australasia.

Boud, D. and Feletti, G. (1997) Changing problem-based learning. Introduction to second edition, in D. Boud and G. Feletti (eds) *The Challenge of Problem Based Learning*, 2nd edn. London: Kogan Page.

Boud, D. and McDonald, R. (1981) *Educational Development through Consultancy*. Guildford: SRHE.

Bowe, B. and Cowan, J. (2004) A comparative evaluation of problem-based learning physics: lecture-based course and a problem-based course, in M. Savin-Baden and K. Wilkie (eds) *Challenging Research in Problem-based Learning*. Maidenhead: SRHE/Open University Press.

Bransford, J.D., Franks, J.J., Vye, N.J. and Sherwood, R.D. (1989) New approaches to instruction: Because wisdom can't be told, in S. Vosniadou and A. Ortany (eds) *Similarity and Analogical Reasoning*. New York: Cambridge University Press.

Braskamp, L.A. and Ory, J.C. (1994) *Assessing Faculty Work: Enhancing Individual and Institutional Performance*. San Francisco: Jossey-Bass.

Brassard, M. (1989) *The Memory Jogger Plus: Featuring the Seven Management and Planning Tools*. Methuen MA: GOAL/QPC.

Bridges, D. (1993) Transferable skills: a philosophical perspective. *Studies in Higher Education*, 18(1): 43–51.

Bridges, E.M. and Hallinger, P. (1996) Problem-based learning in leadership education, in L. Wilkerson and W.H. Gijselaers (eds) *New Directions for Teaching and Learning*. San Francisco: Jossey-Bass, pp. 53–61.

Brookfield, S. (1985) A critical definition of adult education, *Adult Education Quarterly*, 36(1): 44–9.

Brookfield, S. (1994) Tales from the dark side: a phenomenography of adult critical reflection, *International Journal of Lifelong Education*, 13(3): 203–16.

Brookfield, S.D. and Preskill, S. (1999) *Discussion as a Way of Teaching: Tools and Techniques for Democratic Classrooms*. San Francisco: Jossey-Bass.

Brown, S.W., Boyer, M.A., Mayall, H.J., Johnson, P.R., Meng, L., Butler, M.J., Weir, K., Florea, N., Hernandez, M. and Reis, S. (2003) The GlobalEd Project: Gender differences in a problem-based learning environment of international negotiations, *Instructional Science*, 31(4–5): 255–76.

Bruffee, K. (1999) *Collaborative Learning: Higher Education, Interdependence, and the Authority of Knowledge*, 2nd edn. Baltimore and London: The Johns Hopkins University Press.

Cabrera, A.F. (1998) *Collaborative Learning: Preferences, Gains in Cognitive and Affective Outcomes, and Openness to Diversity Among College Students.* Paper presented to Association for the Study of Higher Education, Miami, FL, November.

Cambridge, B. (1996) The paradigm shifts: Examining quality of teaching through assessment of student learning, *Innovative Higher Education*, 20: 287–98.

Camp, M.G. (1996) Problem based learning: A paradigm shift or a passing fad? *Medical Education Online*, 1: 2.

Casey, M.B. and Howson, P. (1993) Educating preservice students based on a problem-centered approach to teaching, *Journal of Teacher Education*, 44: 1–9.

Cashin, W.E. (1990) Student ratings of teaching: Recommendations for use. IDEA Paper No. 22. Center for Faculty Evaluation and Development: Division of Continuing Education, Kansas State University.

Cashin, W.E. (1995) Student ratings of teaching: The research revisited. IDEA Paper No. 32. Center for Faculty Evaluation and Development: Division of Continuing Education, Kansas State University.

Cawley, P. (1997) A problem-based learning module in mechanical engineering, in D. Boud and G. Feletti (eds) *The Challenge of Problem Based Learning*, 2nd edn. London: Kogan Page.

Centra, J.A. (1993) *Reflective Faculty Evaluation: Enhancing Teaching and Determining Faculty Effectiveness.* San Francisco, CA: Jossey-Bass.

Chung, J.C.C. and Chow, S.M.K. (2000) Meeting challenges: Imbedded PBL in large classes, in J. Marsh (ed.) *Implementing Problem-based Learning*, Proceedings of 1st Asia-Pacific Conference on Problem-based Learning, Hong Kong University: Hong Kong, China.

Clark, B. (1980) Academic Culture, working paper no. 42. New Haven, CN: Yale University Higher Education Research Group.

Clarke, R. (1978) The new medical school at Newcastle, New South Wales. *Lancet*, 1: 434–5.

Claxton, G. (2000) The anatomy of intuition in T. Atkinson and G. Claxton (2000) *The Intuitive Practitioner.* Buckingham: SRHE/Open University Press.

Cockrell, K.S., Caplow, J.A.H. and Donaldson, J.F. (2000) A context for learning: Collaborative groups in the problem-based learning environment, *The Review of Higher Education*, 23(3): 347–64.

Coles, C.R. (1985) Differences between conventional and problem-based curricula in their students' approaches to studying, *Medical Education*, 19: 308–9.

Colliver, J. (2000) Effectiveness of problem-based learning curricula: research and theory, *Academic Medicine*, 75: 259–66.

Conway, J. and Little, P. (2000) Adopting PBL as the preferred institutional approach to teaching and learning: Considerations and challenges, *Journal on Excellence in College Teaching*, 11: (2/3) 11–26.

Conway, J., Little, P. and Parker, V. (2000) Cultural Congruence or Cultural Conflict: Challenges in Implementing PBL across Cultures, Proceeding of 2nd Asia Pacific Conference on Problem-based learning. http://www.tp.edu.sg/pblconference/3.htm (accessed 30 July 2003).

Cooper, P.A. (1993) Paradigm shifts in designed instruction: From behaviorism to cognitivism to constructivism, *Educational Technology*, 33(2): 12–18.

Cordeiro, P. and Campbell, B. (1996) Increasing the transfer of learning through problem based learning in educational administration. ERIC Document Reproduction Service No. ED 396 434.

Cox, C.A. (1996) Student responses to problem-based learning in the Caribbean. Paper presented to the meeting of Research in Medical Education. Association of American Medical Colleges, San Francisco, California. April.

Cox, R., Kontianen, S., Rea, N. and Robinson, S. (1981) *Learning and Teaching: An Evaluation of a Course for Teachers in General Practice.* London: University Teaching Methods Unit, Institute of Education.

Curet, M.J. and Mennin, S.P. (2003) The effects of long term vs short term tutors on the quality of the tutorial process and student performance, *Advances in Health Sciences Education*, 8(2): 117–26.

Custer, R.L. (1994) *Performance-Based Education Implementation Handbook.* Columbia, MO: Instructional Materials Lab, University of Missouri.

Dahlgren, M.A., Castensson, R. and Dahlgren, L.O. (1998) PBL from the teachers' perspective, *Higher Education*, 36(4): 437–47.

Das Carlo, M., Swadi, H. and Mpofu, D. (2003) Medical students perceptions of factors affecting productivity of problem-based learning tutorial groups: Does culture influence the outcome? *Teaching and Learning in Medicine*, 15(1): 59–64.

Davies, P. (2000) Approaches to evidence based teaching, *Medical Teacher*, 22(1): 14–21.

Davison and Ward (1999) *Leading International Teams.* Maidenhead: McGraw Hill.

Dawkins, R. (1990) The Selfish Gene: Oxford: Oxford Press.

De Grave, W.S., Dolmans, D.H.J.M. and van der Vleuten, C.P.M. (1998) Tutor intervention profile: reliability and validity, *Medical Education*, 32(3): 262–8.

De Grave, W.S., Dolmans, D.H.J.M. and van der Vleuten, C.P.M. (1999) Profiles of effective tutors in problem-based learning: scaffolding students learning, *Medical Education*, 33(12): 901–96.

de Vries, M., Schmidt, H.G. and de Graaf, E. (1989) Dutch comparisons: cognitive and motivational effects of problem-based learning on medical students, in H.G. Schmidt., M. Lipkin., M.W. de Vries and J.M. Greep (eds) *New Directions for Medical Education.* New York: Springer-Verlag.

Del Mar, C.B. (1997) Training GPs in Problem-based Learning, in J. Conway, R. Fisher, L. Sheridan-Burns, and G. Ryan (eds) *Research and Development in Problem Based Learning: Integrity, Innovation, Integration*, 4: 110–13.

Delanty, G. (2001) *Challenging Knowledge. The University in the Knowledge Society.* Buckingham: SRHE/Open University Press.

Denzin, D. (1989) *Interpretive Interactionism.* London: Sage.

Des Marchais, J.E. (1993) A student-centered, problem-based curriculum: 5 years experience. *Canadian Medical Association Journal*, 148(9): 1567–72.

Dewey, J. (1938) *Experience and Education.* New York: Collier and Kappa Delta Pi.

Dolmans, D.H.J.M., Wolfhagen, I.H.A.P. and Snellen-Balendong, H.A.M. (1994a) Improving the effectiveness of tutors in problem-based learning, *Medical Teacher*, 16(4): 369–77.

Dolmans, D.H.J.M., Wolfhagen, I.H.A.P., Schmidt, H.G. and Van der Vleuten, C.P.M. (1994b) A rating scale for tutor evaluation in a problem-based curriculum: validity and reliability, *Medical Education*, 28(6): 550–8.

Donner, R.S. and Bickley, H. (1993) Problem-based learning in American medical education: an overview, *Bulletin of Medical Library Association*, 81: 294–8.

Drinan, J. (1991) The limits of problem-based learning, in D. Boud and G. Feletti (eds) *The Challenge of Problem Based Learning.* London: Kogan Page.

Duch, B., Groh, S. and Allen, D. (eds) (2001) *The Power of Problem-based Learning.* Sterling, VA: Stylus.

Duek, J.L.E. (2000) Whose group is it anyway? Equity of student discourse in problem-based learning, in D.H. Evensen and C.E. Hmelo (eds) *Problem-based Learning. A Research Perspective.* Mahwah, New Jersey: Lawrence Erlbaum Associates.

Ebenezer, C. (1993) User survey conducted at the Medical Library of the University of Limburg at Maastricht. Technical report, Medical Library, University of Limburg. http://dlist.sir.arizona.edu/archive/00000242/ (accessed 15 September 2003).

Eggins, H. and Macdonald, R. (eds) (2003) *The Scholarship of Academic Development.* Maidenhead: SRHE/Open University Press.

Ellis, W.D. (1938) *A Source Book of Gestalt Psychology.* New York: Harcourt, Brace and World.

Eng, K.H. (2000) Can Asians do PBL? Centre for development of teaching and learning newsletter 3(3): 1–2.

Entwistle, N.J. (1981) *Styles of Learning and Teaching.* New York: John Wiley and Sons Ltd.

Entwistle, N.J. (1987) A model of the teaching-learning process, in R.T.E. Richardson, M.W. Eysenck and D.W. Piper (eds) *Student Learning.* Buckingham: SRHE/Open University Press.

Entwistle, N.J., Hanley, M. and Hounsell, D. (1979) Identifying distinctive approaches to studying, *Higher Education,* 8: 365–80.

Eva, K.W., Neville, A.J. and Norman, G.R. (1998) Exploring the etiology and content specificity: Factors influencing analogic transfer and problem solving, *Academic Medicine,* (73)10: S1–5.

Evensen, D.H. and Hmelo, C.E. (eds) (2000) *Problem-based Learning. A Research Perspective.* Mahwah, New Jersey: Lawrence Erlbaum Associates.

Farmer, D. (1999) Course-embedded assessment: A catalyst for realizing the paradigm shift from teaching to learning, *Journal of Staff, Program and Organizational Development,* 16(4): 199–211.

Fischetti, J., Dittmer, A. and Kyle, D.W. (1996) Shifting paradigms: Emerging issues for educational policy and practice, *Teacher Educator,* 31(3): 189–201.

Fisher, K. (1999) *Leading Self-Directed Work Teams,* 2nd edn. Maidenhead: McGraw-Hill.

Flexner, A. (1910) *Medical Education in the United States and Canada.* Boston: Merrymount Press.

Freire, P. (1972) *Pedagogy of the Oppressed.* London: Penguin Books.

Freire, P. (1974) *Education: The Practice of Freedom.* London: Writers and Readers Publishing Cooperative.

Fuhrmann, B.S. (1996) Philosophies and aims, in J.G. Gaff, J.L. Ratcliff and Associates (eds) *Handbook of the undergraduate curriculum: A comprehensive guide to purposes, structures, practices, and change.* San Francisco: Jossey-Bass.

Gagne, R.M. and Dick, W. (1983) Instructional psychology, *Annual Review of Psychology,* 34: 261–95.

Gallagher, S.A. and Stepien, W.J. (1996) Content acquisition in problem-based learning: Depth versus breadth in American studies, *Journal for the Education of the Gifted,* 19: 257–75.

Garrison, D.R. (1993) A cognitive constructivist view of distance education: An analysis of teaching-learning assumptions, *Distance Education,* 14(2): 199–211.

Gibbons, M., Limoges, C., Nowotny, H., Schwarzman, S., Scott, P. and Trow, M.

(1994) *The New Production of Knowledge: The Dynamics of Science and Research in Contemporary Societies.* London: Sage.

Gibbs, G. (1992) *Improving the Quality of Students Learning.* Bristol: Technical and Educational Services.

Gijselaers, W.H. (1997) Effects of contextual factors on tutor behaviour, *Teaching and Learning in Medicine*, 9(2): 116–24.

Gijselaers, W.H. and Schmidt, H.G. (1990) Development and evaluation of a causal model of problem-based learning, in A.M. Nooman, H.G. Schmidt and E. Ezzat (eds) *Innovation in Medical Education. An Evaluation of its Present Status.* New York: Springer.

Gilligan, C. (1979) Woman's place in man's life cycle, *Harvard Educational Review*, 49: 431–46.

Giroux, H. (1999) Towards a postmodern pedagogy, in L.E. Cahoone (ed.) *From Modernism to Postmodernism: An Anthology.* Cambridge: Basil Blackwell, pp. 687–97.

Glew, R.H. (2003) The problem with problem-based medical education: promises not kept, *Biochemistry and Molecular Biology Education*, 31: 52–6.

Good, T.E. and Brophy, J.E. (1986) *Educational Psychology A Realistic Approach*, 3rd edn. Longman Publishing: New York.

Guild, P.B. and Garger, S. (1998) *Marching to Different Drummers.* Alexandria, VA: Association for Supervision and Curriculum Development, ED 426968.

Haggis, T. (2002) Exploring the 'black box' of process: a comparison of theoretical notions of the 'adult leaner' with accounts of post graduate learning experience, *Studies in Higher Education*, 27(2): 207–20.

Hamilton, S.J. (1994) Freedom transformed: toward a developmental model for the construction of collaborative learning environments, in K. Bosworth and S.J. Hamilton (eds) *Collaborative Learning: Underlying Processes and Effective Techniques New Directions for Teaching and Learning*, 59. San Francisco: Jossey-Bass, pp. 93–101.

Harris, R. (2001) *The Plagiarism Handbook.* Los Angeles: Pyrczak Publishing.

Haslett, L. (2001) McMaster University introduces problem-based learning in medical education, in D. Schugurensky (ed.) *History of Education: Selected Moments of the 20th Century.* http://fcis.oise.utoronto.ca/~daniel_schugurensky/assignment1/1969mcmaster.html (accessed 9 September 2003).

Heredia, A. (1999) Cultural learning styles ERIC Clearinghouse on Teaching and Teacher Education. www.ericcass.uncg.edu/virtuallib/diversity/1036.html (accessed 28 July 2003).

Heron, J. (1989) *The Facilitator's Handbook.* London: Kogan Page.

Heron, J. (1993) *Group Facilitation.* London: Kogan Page.

Hilgard, E.R. and Bower, G.H. (1975) *Theories of Learning*, 4th edn. Englewood Cliffs, NJ: Prentice-Hall Inc.

Hilliard, A.G. III (1988) Behavioral style, culture, teaching and learning. Position paper presented to the New York State Board of Regents' Panel on Learning Styles. Report to New York State Board of Regents' Panel on Learning Styles. New Haven: Yale University Institute for Social and Policy Studies. ED348407.

Holmes, D.B. and Kaufman, D.M. (1994) Tutoring in problem-based learning: a teacher development process, *Medical Education*, 28(4):275–83.

hooks, b. (1989) *Talking Back: Thinking Feminist, Thinking Black.* Boston: South End Press.

Hord, S.M. (1997) Professional learning communities: What are they and why are they important? *Issues . . . about Change* 6(1) http://www.sedl.org/change/issues/issues61.html (accessed on 28 October, 2003).

Hutchings, B. and O'Rourke, K. (2002) Problem-based learning in literary studies, *Arts and Humanities in Higher Education*, 1(1): 73–83.

Hutchings, B and O'Rourke, K. (2004) Medical studies to literary studies: adapting the problem-based learning process for new disciplines, in M. Savin-Baden and K. Wilkie (eds) *Challenging Research 'in Problem-based Learning*. Maidenhead: SRHE/Open University Press.

Irvine, J.J. and York, D.E. (1995) Learning styles and culturally diverse students: a literature review, in J.A. Banks (ed.) *Handbook of Research on Multicultural Education*. New York: Simon and Schuster/Macmillan.

Jacobsen, D.Y. (1997) Tutorial Processes in a Problem-based Learning Context; Medical Students Reception and Negotiations. Unpublished PhD Thesis, Norwegian University of Science and Technology, Norway.

Jaques, D. (2000) *Learning in Groups*, 2nd edn. London: Croom Helm.

Jarvis, P. (1995) *Adult and Continuing Education*, 2nd edn. London: Routledge.

Johnson, D.W., Johnson, R.T. and Smith, K.A. (1991) *Cooperative Learning: Increasing College Faculty Instructional Productivity*. ASHE-ERIC Higher Education Report 4. Washington, DC: The George Washington University, School of Education and Social Development.

Johnson, D.W., Johnson, R.T. and Smith, K.A. (1998) *Active Learning: Cooperation in the College Collaborative Learning Classroom*. Edina, MN: Interaction Book Company.

Jones, R., Higgs, R., de Angelis, C. and Prideaux, D. (2001) Medical education: Changing face of medical curricula, *Lancet*, 357: 699–703.

Kandlbinder, P. and Mauffette, Y. (2001) Perceptions of teaching by science teachers using a students-centred approach, in P. Little and P. Kandbinder (eds) *The Power of Problem-based Learning*. Proceedings of the 3rd Asia Pacific Conference on Problem-based learning.

Kant, I. (1983) *Perpetual Peace and Other Essays on Politics and Morals*. Indianapolis, Indiana: Hackett Publishing Company Inc.

Karmel, P. (1973) Expansion of medical education: report of the committee on medical schools to the Australian Universities Commission. Canberra: Australian Government Publishing Service (AGPS).

Katz, G. (1995) Facilitation, in C. Alavi (ed.) *Problem-based Learning in a Health Sciences Curriculum*. London: Routledge.

Kaufman, D.M. and Holmes, D.B. (1998) The relationship of tutors' content expertise to interventions and perceptions in a problem-based learning medical curriculum, *Medical Education*, 32(3) 255–61.

Khoo, H.E. (2003) Implementations of problem-based learning in Asian medical schools and students perceptions of their experience, *Medical Education*, 37(5): 401–9.

King, S. (2001) Problem-based induction program for first year students. Paper presented to The Power of Problem-based Learning. 3rd Asia Pacific Conference on Problem-based Learning, 9–12 December.

Kippers, V., Price, D. and Isaacs, G. (1997) An Evaluation of Problem-based Learning (PBL) Facilitator Training Program, in J. Conway, R. Fisher, L. Sheridan-Burns, and G. Ryan (eds) *Research and Development in Problem Based Learning Integrity, Innovation, Integration*, 4. Newcastle, Australia: PROBLARC, 262–74.

Kneale, P. (1997) The rise of the 'strategic students': how can we adapt to cope?, in S. Armstrong, G. Thompson and S. Brown (eds) *Facing up to Radical Change in Universities and Colleges*. London: Kogan Page.

Knowles, M. (1978) *The Adult Learner: a Neglected Species.* Houston, Texas: Gulf Publishing Company.

Knowles, M. and Associates (1984) *Andragogy in Action.* San Francisco: Jossey-Bass.

Kolb, D.A. and Fry, R. (1975) Towards an Applied Theory of Experiential Learning, in C.L. Cooper (ed.) *Theories of Group Processes.* Chichester: John Wiley and Sons Ltd.

Koschmann, T., Glenn, P. and Conlee, M. (1997) Analyzing the Emergence of a Learning Issue in a Problem-based Learning Meeting, *Medical Education Online* (2): 2 http://www.utmb.edu/meo/ (accessed 18 October 2003).

Kuh, G.D. and Whitt, E.J. (1988) *The Invisible Tapestry: Culture in American Colleges and Universities,* ASHE-ERIC Higher Education Report, 7(1). Washington, DC: The George Washington University, Graduate School of Education and Human Development.

Land, R. (2003) Orientations to Academic Development, in H. Eggins, and R. Macdonald (eds) *The Scholarship of Academic Development.* Buckingham: SRHE/ Open University Press, 34–46.

Lave, J. and Wenger, E. (1991) *Situated Learning: Legitimate Peripheral Participation.* Cambridge and New York: Cambridge University Press.

Levine, H.G. and Forman, P.B. (1973) A study of retention of knowledge of neurosciences information, *Journal of Medical Education,* 48(9): 867–9.

Lieux, E.M. (1996) A comparative study of learning in lecture versus problem-based format, *About Teaching,* 50: 25–7.

Lincoln, Y.S. and Guba, E.G. (1985) *Naturalistic Inquiry.* Beverly Hills, CA: Sage Publishing.

Lindblom-Ylänne, S., Pihlajamäki, H. and Kotkas, T. (2003) What makes a students group successful? Student-student and student-teacher interaction in a problem-based learning environment, *Learning Environments Research,* 6(1): 59–76.

Little, S. (1997) Preparing Tertiary Teachers for Problem-based Learning, in D. Boud and G. Feletti (eds) *The Challenge of Problem Based Learning,* 2nd edn. London: Kogan Page.

McDaniel, T.R. (1994) College classrooms of the future: Megatrends to paradigm shifts, *College Teaching,* 1(42): 27–31.

Macdonald, R. and Savin-Baden, M. (2003) *A Briefing on Assessment in Problem-based Learning.* LTSN Generic Centre Assessment Series, no. 7. York: LTSN Generic Centre.

McGill, I. and Beaty, L. (2001) *Action Learning,* 2nd edn. London: Kogan Page.

MacGregor, J. (1990) Collaborative learning: Shared inquiry as a process of reform, *New Directions for Teaching and Learning,* 42: 19–30.

McInnis, C. (2000) Changing academic work roles: The everyday realities challenging qualities in teaching, *Quality in Higher Education,* 6(2): 143–53.

McKeachie, W.J. (ed.) (1994) *Teaching Tips,* 9th edn. Lexington, Mass: D.C. Heath and Co.

MacKinnon, M. (1999) PBL in Hong Kong: Three Approaches to Curriculum Reform, PBL Insight, 2(2): 1–6 http://www.samford.edu/pbl/ (accessed 20 August 2003).

Major, C.H. (1999) Connecting what we know and what we do through problem-based learning, *American Association for Higher Education Bulletin,* 51(7): 7–9.

Major, C.H. and Palmer, B. (2002) Faculty knowledge of influences on student learning, *The Peabody Journal of Education,* 77(3): 137–61.

Malantschuk, G. (1971) *Kierkegaard's Thought.* Princeton: Princeton University Press.

Margetson, D. (1991) Is there a future for problem-based education? *Higher Education Review*, 23(2): 33–47.

Margetson, D. (1994) Current educational reform and the significance of problem-based learning, *Studies in Higher Education*, 19(1): 5–19.

Margetson, D. (1997) Wholeness and educative learning: the question of problems in changing to problem-based learning. Keynote speech presented to Changing to Problem-based learning Conference, Brunel University, UK, September.

Marton, F. and Säljö, R. (1976a) On qualitative differences in learning: I. Outcome and process, *British Journal of Educational Psychology*, 46: 4–11.

Marton, F. and Säljö, R. (1976b) On qualitative differences in learning: II. Outcome as a function of the learner's conception of the task, *British Journal of Educational Psychology*, 46: 115–27.

Marton, F. and Säljö, R. (1984) Approaches to learning, in F. Marton, D. Hounsell and N.J. Entwistle (eds) *The Experience of Learning*. Edinburgh: Scottish Academic Press.

Maslow, A.H. (1968) *Towards a psychology being*, 2nd edn. New York: D. Van Nostrand Company.

Matthews, R.S. (1995) Collaborative learning: Creating knowledge with students, in R.H. Menges, M. Weimer and Associates (eds) *Teaching on Solid Ground: Using Scholarship to Improve Practice*. San Francisco: Jossey-Bass.

Maxwell, R. (1998) *21 Irrefutable Laws of Leadership*. Nashville, TN: Thomas Nelson.

Mennin, S.P. and Martinez-Burrola, N. (1990) The cost of problem-based vs. traditional medical education, *Medical Education*, 20(30): 187–94.

Merriam, S. (2001) *The New Update on Adult Learning Theory*. San Francisco, CA: Jossey-Bass.

Mezirow, J. (1981) A critical theory of adult learning and education, *Adult Education*, 32: 3–24.

Millar, S.B. (1999) Learning Through Evaluation, Adaptation, and Dissemination: The LEAD Center, *AAHE Bulletin*, 51(8): 7–9.

Miller, C.M.L. and Parlett, M. (1974) *Up to the Mark: A Study of the Examination Game*. London: Society for Research into Higher Education.

Miller, G.A. (1956) The magical number seven, plus or minus two: Some limits on our capacity for processing information, *Psychological Review*, 63: 81–97. http://www.well.com/user/smalin/miller.html (accessed 10 September 2003).

Millis, B.J. and Cottell, P.G. (1998) *Cooperative Learning for Higher Education Faculty*. Phoenix: Oryx Press.

Mocker, D.W. and Spear, G.E. (1982) Lifelong learning: Formal, nonformal, informal, and self-directed. Information Series No. 241. Columbus: ERIC Clearinghouse on Adult, Career, and Vocational Education, The National Center for Research in Vocational Education, The Ohio State University. (ERIC Document Reproduction Service No. ED 220 723).

Moore, G.A. (1999) *Crossing the Chasm*, 2nd edn. Oxford: Capstone Publishing.

Moore, G.T., Block, S.D., Briggs Style, C. and Mitchell, R. (1994) The influence of the New Pathway curriculum on Harvard medical students, *Academic Medicine*, 69: 983–9.

Mpofu, D.J.S, Das, M., Stewart, T., Dunn, E. and Schmidt, H.G. (1998) Perceptions of group dynamics in problem-based learning session: a time to reflect on group issues, *Medical Teacher*, (20)5: 421–7.

Murray, I. and Savin-Baden, M. (2000) Staff development in problem-based learning, *Teaching in Higher Education*, 5(1): 107–26.

Musal, B., Abacioglu, H., Dicle, O., Akalin, E., Sarioglu, S. and Esen, A. (2002) Faculty development program in Dokuz Eylul School of Medicine: In the process of curriculum change from traditional to PBL, *Medical Education Online* 7(2) www.med-ed-online.org (accessed 5 May 2002).

Nayer, M. (1995) Faculty development for problem-based learning programs, *Teaching and Learning in Medicine*, 7(3): 138–48.

Neville, A.J. (1999) The problem-based learning tutor: Teacher? Facilitator? Evaluator?, *Medical Teacher*, 21(4): 393–401.

Newble, D.I. and Clarke, R.M. (1986) The approaches to learning of students in a traditional and an innovative problem-based medical school, *Medical Education*, 20: 267–73.

Newell, A., Shaw, J.C. and Simon, H.A. (1958) Chess-playing programs, and the problem of complexity, IBM *Journal of Research and Development*, 2(4): 320–35.

Nolte, J., Eller, P. and Ringel, S.P. (1988) Shifting toward problem-based learning in a medical school neurobiology course, *Proceedings of the Annual Conference on Research in Medical Education*, 27: 66–71.

Norman, G.R. and Schmidt, H.G. (1992) The psychological basis of problem-based learning: A Review of the evidence, *Academic Medicine*, 67(9): 557–65.

Ojanlatva, A., Vandenbussche, C., Hedt, H., Horte, A., Haggblorn, T.M., Keron, J., Kahkonene, J., Mottonen, M., Saraste, A. and Turenen, T. (1997) The use of problem-based learning in dealing with cultural minority groups, *Patient Education and Counseling*, 31(2): 171–6.

Oliffe, J. (2000) Facilitation in PBL – espoused theory versus theory in use. Reflections of a first time user. *Australian Electronic Journal of Nursing Education* 5(2) www.Scu.edu.ac/schools/nhcp/aejne/vol-5.oliffejvol5_2.html (accessed 5 May 2001).

Orenstein, P. in association with the American Association of University Women (1994) *School Girls: Young Women, Self-esteem, and the Confidence Gap*. New York: Doubleday.

Painvin, C., Neufeld, V., Norman, G., Walker, I. and Whelan, G. (1979) The 'triple jump' exercise: A structured measure of problem-solving and self-directed learning'. Proceedings of the 18th Annual Conference on Research in Medical Education.

Parlett, M. and Dearden, G. (eds) (1977) *Introduction to Illuminative Evaluation: Studies in Higher Education*. California: Pacific Soundings Press.

Pask, G. (1976) Styles and strategies of learning, *British Journal of Educational Psychology*, 46: 128–48.

Patton, M.Q. (1991) Beyond evaluation myths, *Adult Learning*, 3(2): 9–10.

Perry, W.G. (1970) *Forms of Intellectual and Ethical Development During the College Years: A Scheme*. New York: Holt, Rinehart and Winston.

Perry, W.G. (1988) Different worlds in the same classroom, in P. Ramsden (ed.) *Improving Learning. New Perspectives*. London: Kogan Page.

Piaget, J. (1929) *The Child's Conception of the World*. London: Routledge and Kegan Paul.

Plato. *The Republic of Plato* (trans Francis MacDonald Cornford). London, Oxford: Oxford University Press, 1980.

Popper, K.R. (1970) Normal science and its dangers, in I. Lakatos and A. Musgrave (eds) *Criticisms and the Growth of Knowledge*. Cambridge: Cambridge University Press.

Powles, A., Wintrip, N., Neufeld, V., Wakefield, J., Coates, G. and Burrows, J. (1981)

The 'triple jump' exercise: Further studies of an evaluative technique. Proceedings of the 20th Annual Conference on Research in Medical Education.

Ramsden, P. (1984) The Context of Learning, in F. Marton, D. Hounsell and N.J. Entwistle (eds) *The Experience of Learning*. Edinburgh: Scottish Academic Press.

Ramsden, P. (1991) A performance indicator of teaching quality in higher education: The Course Experience Questionnaire, *Studies in Higher Education*, 16: 129–50.

Ramsden, P. (1992) *Learning to Teach in Higher Education*. London: Routledge.

Rankin, J. (1992) Problem-based medical education: Effect on library use, *Bulletin of the Medical Library Association*, 80(1): 36–43.

Revans, R.W. (1983) *ABC of Action Learning*. Bromley: Chartwell Bratt.

Reynolds, F. (2003) Initial experiences of interprofessional problem-based learning: a comparison of male and female students' views, *Journal of Interprofessional Care*, 17(1): 35–44.

Ritzer, G. (1996) McUniversity in the postmodern consumer society. *Quality in Higher Education*, 2(3): 185–99.

Rogers, C. (1983) *Freedom to Learn for the '80's*. Columbus, Ohio: Merrill.

Rogers, E.M. (1962) *Diffusion of Innovations*. New York: The Free Press.

Rothkopf, E.Z. (1970) The concept of mathemagenic activities, *Review of Educational Research*, 40: 325–36.

Ryan, G. (1997) Promoting educational integrity in PBL programs – choosing carefully and implementing wisely, in J. Conway, R. Fisher, L. Sheridan-Burns and G. Ryan (eds) *Research and Development in Problem Based Learning Integrity, Innovation, Integration*, 4: 564–59.

Sadker, M. and Sadker, D. (1994) *Failing at Fairness: How Our Schools Cheat Girls*. New York: Simon and Schuster.

Savery, J.R. and Duffy, T.M. (1994) Problem based learning: An instructional model and its constructivist framework, *Educational Technology*, 35(5): 31–8.

Savin-Baden, M. (1996) Problem-based learning: a catalyst for enabling and disabling disjunction prompting transitions in learner stances? Unpublished PhD Thesis. University of London Institute of Education.

Savin-Baden, M. (2000) *Problem-based Learning in Higher Education: Untold Stories*. Buckingham: SRHE/Open University Press.

Savin-Baden, M. (2003) *Facilitating Problem-based Learning: Illuminating perspectives*. Buckingham: SRHE/Open University Press.

Schein, E.H. (1985) *Organizational Culture and Leadership: A Dynamic View*. San Francisco: Jossey-Bass.

Schmidt, H.G. (1994) Resolving inconsistencies in tutor expertise research: Does lack of structure cause students to seek tutor guidance, *Academic Medicine*, 69: 656–62.

Schmidt, H.G. and Bouhuijs, P.A. (1980) *Instruction in Task-orientated Groups*. Utrecht, The Netherlands: Het Spectrum.

Schmidt, H.G., Dauphinee, W.D. and Patel, V.L. (1987) Comparing the effects of problem-based and conventional curricula in an international sample, *Journal of Medical Education*, 62: 305–15.

Schmidt, H.G. and Moust, J. (2000a) Towards a taxonomy of problems used in problem-based learning curricula, *Journal on Excellence in College Teaching*, 11(2/3): 57–72.

Schmidt, H.G. and Moust, J. (2000b) Factors affecting small-group tutorial learning: a review of research, in D.H. Evensen and C.E. Hmelo (eds) *Problem-based Learning. A Research Perspective*. Mahwah, New Jersey: Lawrence Erlbaum Associates.

Schoenfeld, A.H. (1985) *Mathematical Problem Solving*. New York: Academic Press.

Schwartz, P. and Webb, G. (1993) *Case Studies in Teaching in Higher Education.* London: Kogan Page.

Scriven, M. (1972) Pros and cons about goal-free evaluation. *Evaluation Comment,* 3(4): 1–4.

Silen, C. (2001) Between Chaos and Cosmos – A driving force for responsibility and independence in learning, in P. Little and P. Kandbinder (eds) The Power of Problem-based Learning. Proceedings of the 3rd Asia Pacific Conference on Problem-based Learning. 128–35.

Slavin, R.E. (1990) *Cooperative Learning: Theory, Research, and Practice.* Boston: Allyn and Bacon.

Stake, R.E. (1978) The case study method in social inquiry, *Educational Researcher,* 7(2): 5–8.

Stark, J.S. and Lattuca, L.R. (1997) *Shaping the College Curriculum: Academic Plans in Action.* Boston: Allyn and Bacon.

Stendahl, B.K. (1976) *Soren Kierkegaard.* Boston: Twayne Publishers.

Stronach, I., Corbin, B., McNamara, O., Stark, S. and Warne, T. (2002) Towards an uncertain politics of professionalism: teacher and nurse identities in flux, *Journal of Educational Policy,* 17(1): 109–38.

Students Online in Nursing Integrated Curricula (SONIC) www.uclan.ac.uk/sonic (accessed 21 October 2003).

Stufflebeam, D.L. (2000) The CIPP model for evaluation, in D.L. Stufflebeam, G.F. Madaus and T. Kellaghan (eds) *Evaluation Models,* 2nd edn. Boston: Kluwer Academic Publishers.

Taylor, M. (1986) Learning for self-direction in the classroom: The pattern of a transition process, *Studies in Higher Education,* 11(1): 55–72.

The Boyer Commission on Educating Undergraduates (1998) *Reinventing Undergraduate Education: A Blueprint for America's Research Universities.* Stony Brook, State University of New York: http://naples.cc.sunysb.edu/Pres/boyer.nsf/ (accessed on 28 October 2003).

Tierney, W.G. and Rhoads, R.A. (1994) Faculty Socialization as Cultural Process: a Mirror of Institutional Commitment. ASHE-ERIC Higher Education Report No. 93–6. Washington DC: The George Washington University.

Tolman, E.C. (1948) Cognitive maps in rats and men, *Psychological Review,* 55: 189–208.

Treisman, P.U. (1985) Study of the mathematics performance of Black students at the University of California, Berkeley (Doctoral dissertation, University of California, Berkeley, 1986), *Dissertation Abstracts International,* 47, 1641–A.

Turpie, I. and Blumberg, P. (1999) Learning by tutoring, *Academic Medicine,* 74(10): 1051–2.

Tyler, R. (1969 [1949]). *Basic Principles of Curriculum and Instruction.* Chicago: University of Chicago Press.

Usher, R. and Edwards, R. (1994) *Postmodernism and Education.* London: Routledge.

Venkatesh, A. (1995) Ethnoconsumerism: a new paradigm to study cultural and cross-cultural consumer behavior, in J.A. Costa and G.J. Bamossy (eds) Marketing in a Multicultural World, Thousand Oaks, CA: Sage.

Vernon, D.T.A. and Blake, R.L. (1993) Does problem-based learning work? A meta-analysis of evaluative research, *Academic Medicine,* 68(7): 550–63.

Virtanen, P.J., Kosunen, E., Holmberg-Marttila, D. and Virjo, I. (1999) What happens in PBL tutorial sessions? Analysis of medical students' written accounts, *Medical Teacher,* 21(3): 270–6.

Vygotsky, L.S. (1978) *Mind in Society: The Development of Higher Psychological Processes.* Cambridge, MA: Harvard University Press.

Walton, H.J. and Mathews, M.B. (1989) Essentials of problem-based learning, *Medical Education,* 23: 542–58.

Webb, G. (1996) *Understanding Staff Development.* Buckingham: SRHE/Open University Press.

Wee, K.N.L. and Kek, Y.C. (2002) *Authentic Problem-based Learning.* Singapore: Prentice Hall.

Wertheimer, M. (1923) Laws of organization in perceptual forms. First published as Untersuchungen zur Lehre von der Gestalt II, in *Psycologische Forschung, 4,* 301–50. Translation published in W. Ellis (1938) *A Source Book of Gestalt Psychology* (pp. 71–88). London: Routledge and Kegan Paul. http://psy.ed.asu.edu/~classics/Wertheimer/Forms/forms.htm (accessed 10 September 2003).

Wertheimer, M. (1959) *Productive Thinking,* enlarged edn. New York: Harper and Row.

Wetzel, M.S. (1996) Developing the role of the tutor/facilitator, *Postgraduate Medical Journal,* 72: 474–7.

White, H.B. (2003) Making problem-based medical education work, *Biochemistry and Molecular Biology Education,* 31: 188–9.

Wilkerson, L., Hafler, J.P. and Lui, P.A. (1991) Case study of student-directed discussion in four problem-based learning tutorial groups, in Research in medical education. Proceedings of the 30th annual conference, *Academic Medicine,* 66: S79–81.

Wilkerson, L. and Hundert, E.M. (1997) Becoming a problem-based tutor: increasing self-awareness through faculty development, in D. Boud and G. Feletti (eds) *The Challenge of Problem Based Learning,* 2nd edn. London: Kogan Page.

Wilkie, K. (2002) Action, attitudes and attributes: developing facilitation skills for problem-based learning. Unpublished PhD Thesis, Coventry University.

Winn, S. (2002) Student motivation: a socio-economic perspective, *Studies in Higher Education,* 27(4): 445–57.

Winter, R., Buck, A. and Sobiechowska, P. (1999) *Professional Experience and the Investigative Imagination.* London: Routledge.

Woods, D.R., Wright, J.D., Hoffman, T.W., Swartman, R.K., Doig, I.D. (1975) Teaching Problem-solving Skills. *Engineering Education,* (1)1: 238. Washington, DC: The American Society for Engineering Education.

Woods, D. (2000) Helping your students gain the most from PBL, in O.S. Tan, P. Little, S.Y. Hee and J. Conway (eds) *Problem-Based Learning: Educational Innovation across Disciplines,* Singapore: Temasek Centre for Problem-Based Learning.

Woodward, C. (1997) What can we learn from programme evaluation studies in medical education, in D. Boud and G. Feletti (eds) *The Challenge of Problem Based Learning,* 2nd edn. London: Kogan Page.

Woodward, C.A. and Ferrier, B.M. (1982) Perspectives of graduates two or five years after graduation from a three-year medical school, *Journal of Medical Education,* 57: 294–302.

Zimitat, C. and Miflin, B. (2003) Using assessment to induct students and staff into the PBL tutorial process, *Assessment and Evaluation in Higher Education,* 28(1): 17–32.

Index

The Society for Research into Higher Education

The Society for Research into Higher Education (SRHE), an international body, exists to stimulate and coordinate research into all aspects of higher education. It aims to improve the quality of higher education through the encouragement of debate and publication on issues of policy, on the organization and management of higher education institutions, and on the curriculum, teaching and learning methods.

The Society is entirely independent and receives no subsidies, although individual events often receive sponsorship from business or industry. The Society is financed through corporate and individual subscriptions and has members from many parts of the world. It is an NGO of UNESCO.

Under the imprint *SRHE & Open University Press*, the Society is a specialist publisher of research, having over 80 titles in print. In addition to *SRHE News*, the Society's newsletter, the Society publishes three journals: *Studies in Higher Education* (three issues a year), *Higher Education Quarterly* and *Research into Higher Education Abstracts* (three issues a year).

The Society runs frequent conferences, consultations, seminars and other events. The annual conference in December is organized at and with a higher education institution. There are a growing number of networks which focus on particular areas of interest, including:

Access	FE/HE
Assessment	Graduate Employment
Consultants	New Technology for Learning
Curriculum Development	Postgraduate Issues
Eastern European	Quantitative Studies
Educational Development Research	Student Development

Benefits to members

Individual

- The opportunity to participate in the Society's networks
- Reduced rates for the annual conferences
- Free copies of *Research into Higher Education Abstracts*
- Reduced rates for *Studies in Higher Education*

- Reduced rates for *Higher Education Quarterly*
- Free online access to *Register of Members' Research Interests* – includes valuable reference material on research being pursued by the Society's members
- Free copy of occasional in-house publications, e.g. *The Thirtieth Anniversary Seminars Presented by the Vice-Presidents*
- Free copies of *SRHE News* and *International News* which inform members of the Society's activities and provides a calendar of events, with additional material provided in regular mailings
- A 35 per cent discount on all SRHE/Open University Press books
- The opportunity for you to apply for the annual research grants
- Inclusion of your research in the *Register of Members' Research Interests*

Corporate

- Reduced rates for the annual conference
- The opportunity for members of the Institution to attend SRHE's network events at reduced rates
- Free copies of *Research into Higher Education Abstracts*
- Free copies of *Studies in Higher Education*
- Free online access to *Register of Members' Research Interests* – includes valuable reference material on research being pursued by the Society's members
- Free copy of occasional in-house publications
- Free copies of *SRHE News* and *International News*
- A 35 per cent discount on all SRHE/Open University Press books
- The opportunity for members of the Institution to submit applications for the Society's research grants
- The opportunity to work with the Society and co-host conferences
- The opportunity to include in the *Register of Members' Research Interests* your Institution's research into aspects of higher education

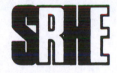

Membership details: SRHE, 76 Portland Place, London
W1B 1NT, UK Tel: 020 7637 2766. Fax: 020 7637 2781.
email: srheoffice@srhe.ac.uk
world wide web: http://www.srhe.ac.uk./srhe/
Catalogue: SRHE & Open University Press, McGraw-Hill
Education, McGraw-Hill House, Shoppenhangers Road,
Maidenhead, Berkshire SL6 2QL. Tel: 01628 502500.
Fax: 01628 770224. email: enquiries@openup.co.uk
web: www.openup.co.uk

Related books from Open University Press
Purchase from www.openup.co.uk or order through your local bookseller

---

FACILITATING PROBLEM-BASED LEARNING
ILLUMINATING PERSPECTIVES

Maggi Savin-Baden

Interest in problem-based learning continues to flourish worldwide. To date there has been relatively little to help staff to examine the complex issues relating to facilitating the implementation of problem-based learning and the ongoing development of staff, students and the curriculum.

This book explores a broad range of issues about facilitation, in particular understandings of facilitation that have emerged from the author's recent research and ways of equipping and supporting staff in terrestrial and virtual contexts. It also questions how students are assessed and suggests ways of preventing plagiarism in problem-based learning. It examines what it might mean to be an effective facilitator and suggests ways of designing problem-based curricula that enhance learning.

Contents

*Acknowledgements – Prologue – **Part one: Re-viewing facilitation** – Perspectives on facilitation – Types and levels of facilitation – **Part two: On becoming a facilitator** – Role transitions: from lecturer to facilitator – Being an effective facilitator – Facilitating honesty in problem-based curricula – **Part three: Facilitation changing worlds** – Developing and supporting facilitators – Virtual facilitation – Beyond surveillance: assessment and facilitation – **Part four: Rhetorical communities** – Reconceptualising problem-based curricula – Facilitating learning in problem-based curricula – Epilogue: Changing places or changing spaces? – Glossary – Bibliography – Index.*

176pp   0 335 21054 6 (Paperback)   0 335 21055 4 (Hardback)

TEACHING FOR QUALITY LEARNING AT UNIVERSITY
SECOND EDITION

John Biggs

> Full of downright good advice for every academic who wants to do something practical to improve his or her students' learning ... there are very few writers on the subject of university teaching who can engage a reader so personally, express things so clearly, relate research findings so eloquently to personal experience.
>
> Paul Ramsden

Since the first edition of *Teaching for Quality Learning at University*, the tertiary sector has changed dramatically. Individual teachers, as reflective practitioners, still need to make their own decisions about how they are going to get students actively involved in large classes, to teach international students, and to assess in ways that enhance the quality of learning. But now that quality assurance and quality enhancement are required at the institutional level, the concept of constructive alignment is applied to 'the reflective institution', where it becomes a powerful underpinning to quality enhancement procedures.

Also since the first edition, educational technology has become more widespread than expected, leaving some teachers apprehensive about what it might mean for them. A new chapter elaborates on how ET can be used to enhance learning, but with a warning that any tool, electronic or otherwise, is as good as the thoughtful use to which it is put.

This is an accessible, jargon-free guide to all university teachers interested in enhancing their teaching and their students' learning, and for administrators and teaching developers who are involved in teaching-related decisions on an institutional basis.

Contents

336pp   0 335 21168 2 (Paperback)   0 335 21169 0 (Hardback)

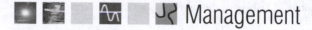
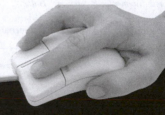
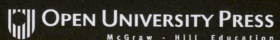